HYPNOSIS, DISSOCIATION, AND ABSORPTION

THEORIES, ASSESSMENT, AND TREATMENT

By

MARTY SAPP, ED.D.

Professor
University of Wisconsin–Milwaukee
Department of Educational Psychology, Counseling Area

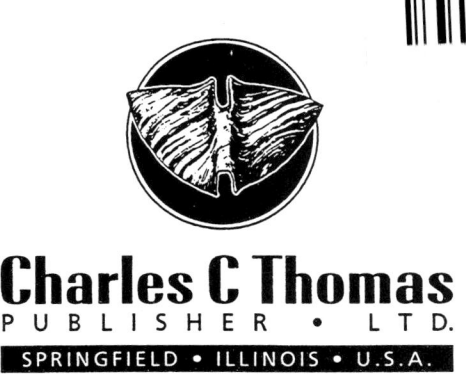

Charles C Thomas
PUBLISHER • LTD.
SPRINGFIELD • ILLINOIS • U.S.A.

Published and Distributed Throughout the World by

CHARLES C THOMAS • PUBLISHER, LTD.
2600 South First Street
Springfield, Illinois 62704

This book is protected by copyright. No part of it may be reproduced in any manner without written permission from the publisher.

©2000 by CHARLES C THOMAS • PUBLISHER, LTD.

ISBN 0-398-07054-7 (cloth)
ISBN 0-398-07055-5 (paper)

Library of Congress Catalog Card Number: 99-086788

With THOMAS BOOKS *careful attention is given to all details of manufacturing and design. It is the Publisher's desire to present books that are satisfactory as to their physical qualities and artistic possibilities and appropriate for their particular use.* THOMAS BOOKS *will be true to those laws of quality that assure a good name and good will.*

Printed in the United States of America
JS-R-3

Library of Congress Cataloging-in-Publication Data

Sapp, Marty, 1958-
  Hypnosis, dissociation, and absorption : theories, assessment, and treatment / Marty Sapp.
    p. cm.
  Includes bibliographical references and indexes.
  ISBN 0-398-07054-7 (hardcover) --ISBN 0-398-07055-5 (pbk.)
  1. Hypnotism--Therapeutic use. I. Title.

RC495 .S334 2000
616.89'162--dc21   99-086788

To the students in my clinical hypnosis course and the students of my hypnosis research team.

PREFACE

Hypnosis, Dissociation, and Absorption: Theories, Assessment, and Treatment presents the psychological theories and applications of how to use hypnosis with clients who display dissociation, absorption, fantasy proneness, and imaginative capabilities. This book discusses hypnosis, dissociation, and absorption from a theoretical, assessment, and clinical perspective. Moreover, this text discusses the clinical implications of applying hypnosis to several overlapping psychological disorders such as dissociative identity disorder, borderline personality disorder, somatoform disorder, and posttraumatic stress disorder. In addition, the uses of hypnosis for pain control, anxiety and stress, ego-strengthening, unipolar depression, smoking cessation, weight loss, and rehabilitation are described. Finally, this text provides treatment transcripts including, but not limited to, the following theoretical approaches: cognitive-behavioral, psychodynamic, and Ericksonian.

This text clearly brings together assessment, research, dissociative disorders, and hypnotic treatment in one place. Even though the treatment of dissociative disorders is a widely published area, this book adds to the literature by providing a step-by-step approach to the clinical interview and preparation of the client for hypnosis. Many clinicians will clamor for this specific information. The presentation of verbatim transcripts allow a clinician to employ quality transcripts within a self-teaching format. Finally, this text provides a diversity of topics and a variety of treatment techniques.

M.S.

ACKNOWLEDGMENTS

SEVERAL INDIVIDUALS HELPED BRING THIS TEXT INTO PRESS. First, I would like to thank students in my clinical hypnosis course, especially Ms. Khyána Pumphrey, for proofreading this entire manuscript. Moreover, I would like to thank the students who were members of my hypnosis research teams. Second, I offer thanks to Ms. Cathy Mae Nelson and the University of Wisconsin–Milwaukee School of Education word-processing pool for typing this entire manuscript. I thank Dr. Walter Farrell, the Department of Educational Policy and Community Studies at the University of Wisconsin–Milwaukee, who served as my academic mentor. I offer thanks to my University of Cincinnati connections: Dr. Patricia O'Reilly, Dr. Judith Frankel, Dr. Marvin Berlowitz, Dr. Purcell Taylor, and Dr. James Stevens. I offer special thanks to Dr. David L. Johnson of Xavier University in Cincinnati, who taught me how to embrace the scientist-practitioner model of being a psychologist. Finally, thanks also go to Dr. Cheryl L. Johnson at Miami University of Ohio. In closing, comments or discussions concerning this text–both positive and negative–are encouraged. My address is The University of Wisconsin–Milwaukee, Department of Educational Psychology, 2400 E. Hartford Avenue, Milwaukee, Wisconsin 53211. My telephone number is (414) 229-6347, my e-mail address is sapp@uwm.edu, and my fax number is (414) 229-4939.

CONTENTS

	Page
Preface	vii
Chapter	
1. USES OF HYPNOSIS	3
2. HISTORY OF PSYCHOLOGICAL THEORIES	6
Mesmer and Animal Magnetism	6
Charcot	8
Janet	9
The Nancy School: Liébault and Bernheim	9
Faria	10
De Puységur	11
Coué	11
Braid	12
Phases of Freud's Psychoanalysis	13
Freud and Repression	16
Summary	17
Clinical Applications	18
Discussion Questions	18
3. PHENOMENA OF HYPNOSIS	19
APA's Division 30 Definition of Hypnosis	19
Phenomena of Hypnosis:	19
Absorption and Dissociation	20
Repression	22
Suppression	22
Catalepsy	23
Amnesia and Hyperamnesia	23

Analgesia, Anesthesia, and Hyperesthesia	23
Ideomotor and Ideosensory Exploration	24
Somnambulism	24
Hallucinations	25
Age Regression, Age Progression, and Time Distortion	25
Depersonalization and Derealization	26
Current Theories of Hypnosis	26
Ericksonian Hypnosis	27
Dissociation Theories	29
Cognitive-Behavioral Theories	32
Sociophenomenological Theories	34
Psychological Regression	34
Relaxation Theory of Hypnosis	36
Clinical Applications	37
Discussion Questions	38
4. DISSOCIATIVE DISORDERS	**39**
Borderline Personality Disorder	42
Hypnosis Applications for BPD	45
Overview of Dissociative Identity Disorder (DID):	46
Description of DID	46
Differential Diagnosis and DID	48
Treatment of DID	49
Postfusion Treatment	53
Hypnosis Applications for DID	53
Summary	54
Dissociative Disorders in Children	54
Assessment of Dissociative Disorders in Children	55
Screening Instruments for Dissociative Disorders with Children	57
Chapter Summary	58
5. TREATMENT	**59**

Chapter Overview	59
Preparation of a Client for Hypnosis	59
Hypnotic Screening Tests	61
Handclasp Hypnotic Screening Test Debriefing	62
Hand Levitation Hypnotic Screening Test	63
Debriefing	63
Case Presentation	64
Case Presentation Summary	66
Ingredients of Hypnosis Transcripts	66
Direct Hypnosis	67
Direct Hypnosis Transcript	67
Indirect Hypnosis	69
Indirect Hypnosis Transcript	69
Debriefing	76
Cognitive-Behavioral Hypnosis (CBH)	76
CBH Transcript	76
Debriefing	77
Psychoanalysis and Hypnosis	78
Erika Fromm	78
Michael Nash	79
Psychodynamic Hypnosis Transcript	80
Debriefing	81
Hypnosis Fusion Technique for DID	82
Debriefing	83
Dissociation Transcript	83
Debriefing	85
Age Progression Transcript	85
Age Regression Transcript	86
Debriefing	86
Implications of Hypnosis for Pain Control	87
Pain Control Transcript	88
Debriefing	89
Anxiety and Stress	89
Anxiety and Stress Transcript	89
Debriefing	91

Ego Strengthening Induction Transcript	90
Debriefing	91
Unipolar Depression	91
Unipolar Depression Transcript	92
Debriefing	93
Smoking	93
Smoking Cessation Transcript	94
Debriefing	94
Hypnosis and Weight Loss	94
Hypnosis and Weight Loss Transcript	95
Debriefing	96
Hypnosis and Rehabilitation	96
Rehabilitation Hypnosis Transcript	97
Debriefing	97
Possible Negative Sequelae of Hypnosis	97
Chapter Conclusion	99
6. CONTEMPORARY HYPNOSIS THEORIES AND RESEARCH	**101**
Contemporary Hypnosis Theories and Research	101
Chapter Overview	101
Barber's Paradigm	102
Spanos	103
Hilgard	103
Barber's 3-Dimensional Paradigm	103
Fantasy-Prone	103
The Amnesic Prone	104
The Positively-Set Clients	105
Summary and Conclusions for Research	106
Measures of Hypnotic Responding	108
Hypnotic Depth	109
Hypnotizability Scales Reflecting a Cognitive-Behavioral Orientation	111
Indirect Hypnotic Susceptibility Scale	113
Hypnotizability Measures and Theoretical Perspectives	113

Hypnosis and Memory
Hypnosis, Automaticity, Involuntariness, and
   Nonvolitional Responding   115
Research Instruments   121
   Vividness of Imagination Scale (VIS)   122
   Hypnosis Survey (HS)   122
   Description of Hypnotic Experience   125
   Description of Hypnotic Regression Experience   126
   General Dissociation Scale (GDS)   126
      Table 1: General Dissociation Scale (GDS)   127
      Table 2: Means and Standard Deviations
         of GDS Items   130
      Table 3: Correlation Matrix of GDS Items   131
      Table 4: Principle Components Analysis of
         GDS   132
   Chapter Summary   133

7. PULLING IT TOGETHER: WHAT IS HYPNOSIS AND WHY IS IT RELATED TO DISSOCIATION AND ABSORPTION?   134

References   137
Author Index   153
Subject Index   157

HYPNOSIS, DISSOCIATION, AND ABSORPTION

Chapter 1

USES OF HYPNOSIS

HYPNOSIS IS AN ADJUNCTIVE PROCEDURE that can be used to treat many psychological disorders such as substance-related disorders, mood disorders, anxiety disorders, somatoform disorders, dissociative disorders, sexual disorders, eating disorders, adjustment disorders, attention-deficit disorder, and obsessive-compulsive disorder. For any psychological disorder in which a clinician has training, regardless of his or her theoretical orientation, hypnosis is an adjunctive procedure that can enhance clinical practice. For example, hypnosis has an effect size, a quantitative measure of effectiveness, larger than any other procedure (Sapp 1997b).

In addition, meta-analyses, statistical methods for summarizing several studies, have shown that hypnosis increases the effect sizes of cognitive-behavioral and psychodynamic therapies. Moreover, hypnosis can change clients' expectations, which is probably the ultimate goal of psychotherapy.

Hypnosis is particularly useful for clients who display dissociation, absorption, fantasy proneness, and imaginative capabilities. Clinically, this is one reason why hypnosis is the treatment of choice for several overlapping disorders that have dissociation as the central feature, such as dissociative identity disorder, borderline personality disorder, somatoform disorder, and posttraumatic stress disorder.

Farthing, Venturino, Brown, and Lazar (1997); Chaves and Dworkin (1997); Patterson, Adcock, and Bombardier (1997); Tan and Leucht (1997), Dinges et al. (1997); and Perry, Gelfand, and Marcovitch (1979) found that conditions such as pain, asthma, and warts were moderated by bodily functions that are nonconscious and can be changed by altering clients' perceptions through hypnosis. Moreover, Hilgard and Hilgard (1994) documented how pain relief and hypnosis were related. For example, clients' levels of hypnotizability were directly correlated with the amount of relief received from pain. Specifically, for clients with high levels of hypnotizability, hypnosis produced more analgesic relief than could morphine (Stern, Brown, Ulett & Sletten 1977).

This explains how hypnosis has been used as the sole analgesic in surgeries ranging from tooth extractions to cardiac surgeries. Moreover, hypnosis has been applied to the field of obstetrics. Likewise, hypnosis has been used to reduce pain associated with redressing burn wounds, as well as to reduce migraine headaches, and it has been used to control bleeding during and after surgeries (Morgan & Hilgard 1973; Orne & Dinges 1984). Finally, in terms of psychoanalytic and psychodynamic therapies, hypnosis can be used to facilitate clients' ability to uncover unconscious information, and hypnosis can be used to facilitate transference during the analysis of transference phase of psychotherapy.

The following chapters were established in a hierarchical order. Chapter 2 discusses the early psychological theories of hypnosis that have roots which predate psychoanalysis. Chapter 3 provides a description of the phenomena of hypnosis such as dissociation, absorption, repression, suppression, catalepsy, amnesia, hyperamnesia, analgesia and anesthesia, hyperesthesia, ideomotor and ideomotor exploration, somnambulism, hallucinations, age regression, age progression, time distortion, depersonalization, and derealization. Chapter 4 provides a clinical discussion of the domain of dissociation such as dissociative identity disorder, borderline personality disorder, somatoform disorder, and posttraumatic stress disorder. Chapter 5 describes how to prepare a client for hypnosis, and treatment transcripts are provided for direct hypnosis, indirect hypnosis, cognitive-behavioral hypnosis, psychodynamic hypnosis, cognitive behavioral hypnosis, psychodynamic hypnosis, dissociation, and regression phenomena of hypnosis. Moreover, transcripts are provided for pain control, anxiety and stress, ego strengthening, unipolar depression, smoking cessation, weight loss, and rehabilitation. Chapter 6 provides information on contemporary hypnosis theories and research such as hypnotizability scales, dissociation scales, absorption scales, and hypnosis and memory. Finally, Chapter 7 presents a synthesis concerning the complex meanings of hypnosis, and it concludes by showing why hypnosis, dissociation, and absorption are related.

Chapter 2

HISTORY OF PSYCHOLOGICAL THEORIES

MESMER AND ANIMAL MAGNETISM

DURING THE 16TH CENTURY, a Swiss physician and alchemist, Philippus Paracelsus (1493-1541), rejected the witch-hunts and demon theories of mental illness. Paracelsus believed that a "universal spirit" permeated the world (Hergenhahn 1997, 441), and he believed that magnets, chemicals, and the alignment of stars and other heavenly bodies could influence one's mental and physical health.

Franz Anton Mesmer (1734–1815) continued this evolution of mental illness from supernatural explanations into more psychological explanations. Mesmer, like Paracelsus, believed that the planets influenced humans through a force called *animal gravitation*. This was an analogue to Newton's theory of universal gravitation.

In the early 1770s, Mesmer met Father Maximillian Hell, a priest, who reported curing ailments with magnets. Actually, earlier, Paracelsus and others had used magnets to treat disorders. Mesmer theorized that psychological disorders were the result of a magnetic force (animal magnetism) being unevenly distributed throughout one's body. Theoretically, the goal of Mesmer's approach was to redistribute the animal magnetism which produced an abreaction within the client where he or she would typically scream, perspire, and experience convulsions. Mesmer found that clients' abreactions led to catharsis and a subsiding of the psychophysiological symptoms. It is apparent that many of Mesmer's clients experienced what was called at the time hysterical blindness, paralysis, and other conversion disorders. Mesmer's theory of magnetic fluid was similar to the emerging theory of electricity. It was discovered that electricity could be transferred from one object to another, so Mesmer made the analogous assumption that animal magnetism could be transferred from one person to another or from an object to a person.

Mesmer was known as a showman, and he made many exaggerated claims about his theory and technique. He performed his demonstration in a dark room with a *baquet* or a box or tub with water, powdered glass, iron, and magnets. He believed that this mixture contained magnetic fluid. Mesmer would enter the room wearing a silk robe and holding a long rod. As he played music, he would walk among his clients and touch them with his hands or his rod. Often, he would have additional rods projecting from the baquet so clients could apply them to their painful body parts. Interestingly, Mesmer did not make mesmeric passes over his clients nor was he acquainted with mesmeric sleep (Hadfield 1967, 28).

Mesmer's flamboyant performances ended when the Faculty of Medicine, in Paris in 1831, held a commission which included Benjamin Franklin; Antoine Lavoisier, the famous chemist; and Joseph Guillotin, the creator of a creative and humane way of putting people to death called the guillotine. The commission ruled that animal magnetism did not exist, and the results were the consequences of clients' imaginations. Mesmer was crushed by this observation, and he withdrew from the public limelight.

CHARCOT

Jean Martin Charcot (1825-1893), a renowned neurologist at the Medical School of La Salpêtrière in Paris, greatly influenced hypnosis. He demonstrated that hysteria was a mental disorder of men as well as women and could not be the result of the womb (Hadfield 1967, 42). In 1862, he became director of La Salpêtrière, and during his tenure, he and his colleagues identified abnormalities of the brain and spinal cord, such as poliomyelitis and multiple sclerosis. In addition, he identified a degenerative disease of the motor neurons that is still known as Charcot's disease—multiple sclerosis or insular sclerosis. Moreover, Charot helped identify many brain structures; he instituted temperature monitoring as a daily hospital routine; and Alfred Binet, William James, and Sigmund Freud all studied with Charcot from October 12, 1885, until February 28, 1886 (Hergenhahn 1997, 452).

Due to his medical model and training, Charcot believed that hysteria, like other neurological disorders such as multiple sclerosis, was progressive and irreversible. Furthermore, he believed that hysteria and hypnosis produced the same symptoms; therefore, he concluded that only hysterics could be hypnotized.

Charcot found that many of his hysterical clients had experienced a trauma and hence concluded that trauma caused neurological damage. Likewise, Charcot speculated that traumas could cause certain ideas to become dissociated from conscious experience and thus isolated from conscious thought. There were two aspects to Charcot's theory. First, clients who were hysterical inherited a biological potential for hysteria. Second, trauma caused clients' ideations to dissociate or "split off" from conscious awareness. Freud concluded from Charcot's theory that physiological symptoms could be caused by unconscious psychological disturbances. It should be noted that Freud accepted Charcot's notions uncritically and as facts.

JANET

Pierre Janet (1759-1947), a professor of psychology in Paris, was a student and colleague of Charcot. Janet characterized hysteria as a dissociating or "splitting off" of conscious and unconscious aspects of the personality. Actually, it was Janet who originated the notion of mental dissociation. More specifically, he described hysteria as a form of dissociation in which there was a retraction in consciousness.

Janet's treatment of hysteria involved three phases. First, discover through hypnosis which experiences were forgotten, dissociated, and the causes of hysterical symptoms. Second, he would bring unconscious experiences into consciousness, thus integrating the personality and resolving dissociation. Third, he used hypnotic suggestions to bolster the morale of the client and to increase psychological energy. It is apparent that Janet's method was analytic in that he regressed clients' psyches back to unconscious psychological distress. Because Janet's and Freud's ideas are so similar, there is disagreement over the ownership of these ideas. Watson (1978) stated that Janet argued that Freud's theory of psychoanalysis oriented from the work of Janet and Charcot.

THE NANCY SCHOOL: LIÉBAULT AND BERNHEIM

Liébault (1823-1904) is regarded as the father of therapeutic suggestion. He, like Janet, was a clinician. Liébault used hypnosis for humanitarian purposes to relieve human suffering. For example, he treated the rich and poor, and unlike Mesmer, he was not a showman. Moreover, in contrast to his contemporary, Charcot, he was extremely skilled with hypnosis.

Liébault was helped greatly by Hippolyte Bernheim (1840-1919). Bernheim was a graduate of La Salpêtrière school under Charcot. He turned away from Charcot's theory of hypnosis because it was pathological in nature; it viewed dissociation as the result of a pathology. The Nancy School stressed the suggestibility aspects of hypnosis. Liébault and his major spokesman, Bernheim, believed that hypnosis was a form of suggestion. And they believed that suggestion was an everyday aspect of life. The implications of this position is that theories of hypnosis expanded from abnormal theoretical origins into normal ones. Moreover, another implication of this suggestibility theory of hypnosis is that normal people can be hypnotized through the use of suggestions. Finally, Bernheim demonstrated that hypnosis could affect the dermatological system by having participants produce blisters on their bodies through hypnosis.

Bernheim was the first to point out that suggestions were effective without hypnosis, and he claimed that hypnosis was suggestion (Weitzenhoffer 1976). Bernheim stated, "There is no hypnosis, there is only suggestion." Weitzenhoffer claimed that Bernheim believed that hypnosis was an altered state of awareness. In addition, Bernheim anticipated Janet's dissociation theory of hypnosis. One implication of Bernheim's suggestion theory is that phenomena associated with hypnosis can be produced without the induction of hypnosis. Later, Barber (1969) and Sarbin and Coe (1972) experimentally supported this important implication. Finally, Weitzenhoffer stated that Bernheim believed that hypnosis produced a state of hypersuggestibility.

FARIA

Abbé Faria (1755 or 1756 to 1819) started public demonstrations of animal magnetism in Paris in 1813. He reduced the extensive rituals of the magnetic movement by requesting that participants close their eyes and focus their attention on sleep (Perry 1978). After a short period, Faria would instruct participants with one word: "Sleep." Perry stated that Faria laid the foundations of trait and skills models of hypnosis by documenting individual variability in hypnotic responsiveness. In contrast to the magnetists, he believed that hypnotic responsiveness depended almost entirely on the inherent abilities of the participants. He discounted the

Faculty of Medicine in Paris in 1831 that found the results of hypnosis were produced by clients' imaginations. In contrast to Bernheim, he gave little emphasis to the role of suggestion in explaining hypnosis. Faria thought that hypnosis was the result of participants' ability to concentrate. Faria referred to hypnosis as "lucid sleep." In 1843, Braid used the term hypnosis which is *hypnos* from Greek and means "to sleep." Faria was aware that motivation was important for producing hypnosis, and he was aware of the placebo effects. To summarize, it is clear that many current theories of hypnosis were influenced by Faria; however, often, his contributions are severely underestimated.

DE PUYSÉGUR

Marquis de Puységur (1751-1825) was most likely Mesmer's most famous student; however, he is known for observing "artificial somnambulism" during mesmerism. He believed that hypnosis was a form of mental transference from the magnetist to the client, in contrast to magnetism. De Puységur also believed that clients were clairvoyant and could diagnose their own illnesses, prescribe the nature of treatment, and predict the date they would be cured (Ellenberger 1970). Finally, Puységur thought that hypnosis was associated with clairvoyance.

COUÉ

Emile Coué, born in 1857 in Troyes, Aube, France, popularized the New Nancy School of hypnosis. Between 1885 and 1886, Coué observed Liébault and was so impressed with the auto-suggestive techniques of the New Nancy School that he opened a free clinic in London (Edmonston 1986). Coué and his wife opened another institute near their home in Nancy. Moreover, in 1922, Coué also established an institute in New York City. Coué believed that hypnosis was the result of auto-suggestion, and his methods relied heavily on the powers of the unconscious. This notion is very similar to the principles taught by Milton H. Erickson in the 1950s and 1960s (Edmonston, 181). Coué started many suggestions with "Every day, in every way, you are getting better and better," which is the foundation for John Hartland's ego strengthening techniques. Charles Baudouin, one of Coué's main advocates, kept Coué's ideas popular during the 1920s and 1930s. Earlier, Bernheim had done a similar thing for Liébault. Very similar to the Ericksonian teachings, Coué believed that the best hypnotist communicated with his or her client's unconscious, rather than the conscious frame of reference.

Furthermore, Coué's theory emphasized positive suggestions and health. Clearly, Erickson and Hartland were influenced by Coué's clinical work; however, he failed to clearly distinguish auto-suggestions from suggestibility. Specifically, suggestions are simply the process of communicating ideas, while suggestibility is the client's acceptance of such ideas.

BRAID

James Braid (1795-1860), born in Scotland, was the English successor to Faria. Braid, in 1843, introduced a physiological theory of mesmerism and referred to it as hypnosis or nervous sleep which was derived from the Greek meaning "to sleep." Gravitz (1991) noted that although Braid is generally given credit as the originator of the term hypnosis, this is not the case because others had used similar terminology earlier. Edmonston (1981) expanded explicitly this concept to describe hypnosis as simply relaxation. Braid also stressed the importance of imagination and the client's belief system in producing hypnosis.

PHASES OF FREUD'S PSYCHOANALYSIS

Freud's psychoanalysis has **three** phases, and the term psychoanalysis is used in **three** distinct ways. **First**, let us describe the term psychoanalysis. It is a theory that loosely describes the structure of the mind, the development of personality, and psychopathology. **Second**, it is a technique used to treat a range of psychological difficulties. **Third**, psychoanalysis is a method of scientific investigation. That is, Freud based psychoanalysis on a clinical observation called **case study methodology**. In addition, Freud based psychoanalysis on the chemistry, physics, and the emerging theory of neurons of the 1800s (Sapp 1997).

From its inception, psychoanalysis was viewed as a method of uncovering psychopathological memories and a shift in mentation from nonadaptive patterns to adaptive ones. Furthermore, psychoanalysis has been associated with several mechanisms related to hypnosis such as repression, regression, automaticity, and dissociation. All of these mechanisms will be discussed later within this text.

During the **first phase of psychoanalysis**, Freud found that his clients were capable of mentation that was not immediately accessible to conscious awareness. As one will see in Chapter 6, many behaviors are nonconscious and automatic, especially hypnotically induced responses. And hypnotically induced behaviors feel to the client to be automatic. That is, these responses require few cognitive resources. Hence, humans can perform several behaviors—cooking while talking on the phone, driving and talking—because the human brain requires few mental resources for many human behaviors. In essence, during the first phase of psychoanalysis, Freud found that his clients were capable of nonconscious processes, which he referred to as **unconscious** activities.

Actually, during Freud's earlier theorizing about hypnosis, he viewed hypnosis as the lack of communication between conscious and unconscious mentation. As one will see within a later section of this chapter, Freud thought that repression was the mechanism that allowed clients to forget or push ideas out of consciousness.

The "splitting off," or **dissociation** of mental processes, often symbolically translated into psychophysiological symptoms (hysteria). Freud viewed disorders such as hysteria as being based on a psychological mechanism and not a neurological one.

In summary, during phase one of psychoanalysis, Freud found that the central aspect of human mentation was unconscious thoughts that could be accessed through slips of the tongue, jokes, dreams, fantasies, hypnosis, free association, and so on.

The **second phase of psychoanalysis** started with Freud discarding hypnosis and replacing it with free association. That is, Freud would have a client lie supinely on a couch, with the client in front of him, he would instruct his client to say freely anything that came into conscious awareness, without the use of censorship.

Freud found that **free association** allowed clients to voluntarily suspend conscious censorship and to allow the emergence of repressed or unconscious materials, and he believed that psychoanalysis accounted for transference and resistance within clients. Because Freud wanted a theory that was uniquely his own, he moved away from hypnosis, which was viewed as a mode of therapy, and toward psychoanalysis, and he developed his own specific techniques such as dream analysis, free association, and so on.

With the **final phase of psychoanalysis**, the third phase, Freud elaborated on his notion of dream analysis and primary and secondary processes. **Primary processes** are nonlogical or id associated **mentation**, and they are connected with the pleasure principle. Moreover, primary processes can be found in dreams, poetry, myths and magic, and the ultimate form of primary process—psychosis. Secondary processes are governed by the laws of logic and are associated with the ego and the reality principle. In 1923, Freud wrote *The Ego and the Id*. This consolidated the concepts of primary and secondary processes.

During the latter part of the third phase of psychoanalysis, other analysts, Jung (1875–1961), Adler (1870–1937), Horney (1885–1952), Sullivan (1892–1949), and Erikson (1902–1992) modified Freud's psychoanalysis (Sapp 1997).

Clinically, why is Freud's theory of psychoanalysis important? And, second, why is this theory important to the practice of hypnosis? First, Freud's psychoanalysis has been integrated into American culture and language. For example, it is common for many Americans to search for historical causes (past) of their current behaviors.

Second, the **intrapsychic nature** of Freud's theory of **psychic energy** being sealed within the client's psyche, and it can move to the mouth, anus, and genitals is interesting; however, this notion of psychic energy provides a complex scheme for understanding some of the nonconscious mechanisms of human behavior. Clearly, Freud's original theory was incorrect; however, he was correct when he theorized that much of behavior is nonconscious and automatic. To illustrate, clients may have reasons for their behaviors (nonconscious and automatic) that are not immediately accessible to consciousness.

The major error with Freud's theory was not the emphasis he gave to sex and aggression, but his faulty interpretation of the developing theories of chemistry and physics. Being technically eclectic, the current writer can use procedures and techniques from Freud's psychoanalysis, which can be helpful to clients, without subscribing to the faulty aspects of the theory. Within the broad range of psychoanalytic theories—Jung, Sullivan, Erikson—theories have many epistemologically incompatible constructs. This is why the theoretical integration of these theories is impossible.

Finally, Freud's theory is important to hypnosis because it was developed from theories of hypnosis and from treatments of hysteria. Furthermore, Freud's theory of psychoanalysis allows a clinician to explore many mechanisms of hypnosis such as regression, repression, dissociation, and automaticity. In closing, the next section explores Freud's theory of repression and hypnosis.

FREUD AND REPRESSION

Sigmund Freud (1856-1939) believed that repression was the cornerstone of hypnosis. Freud's notion of repression was clearly influenced by Charcot's and Janet's theories. **Repression** is an expansive construct in that it can be conscious, unconscious, and automatic. Moreover, it can be a general personality orientation and a defense mechanism.

Freud saw repression as the most important mental mechanism and as the cornerstone of psychoanalysis. Repression can be viewed as the active process of pushing an unpleasant idea out of the mind. For example, many reprehensible notions are often repressed, and the effort used during repression often results in psychological disorders. The reason Freud viewed repression as always unconscious is because often we repress experiences that we are not aware that we are repressing; hence, that which is repressed becomes unconscious (Hadfield 1967, 134; Singer 1990). The immediate result of repression is dissociation—or the splitting off of parts of the mind (conscious vs. unconscious). Likewise, repression is the process in which dissociation occurs. When clients split off experiences (affects from sensations or cognitions), the resulting dissociation can produce psychological disorders.

Another confusing notion about repression is that Freud often used repression and dissociation interchangeably; nevertheless, as previously stated, repression is the process through which dissociation occurs. Ideations that are dissociated are referred to as complexes, or experiences that are incompatible with the personality, and are repressed and dissociated from the mind. Complexes are emotionally charged ideations that are unconscious, because one is not aware of them. Finally, repression can give rise to a host of defense mechanisms such as overcompensation, projection, introjection, displacement, regression, rationalization, and so on.

During 1880, Josef Breuer (1842–1925) found what Charcot and Janet had discovered earlier: that hypnosis facilitated catharsis and helped in uncovering traumatic memories. Freud was trained in hypnosis by Breuer and Bernheim at the Nancy School; however, Freud only dabbled in hypnosis, and he did not find it helpful with difficult cases. Freud became even more disenchanted with hypnosis when a female client leaped upon him in a romantic way during hypnosis. Because Freud viewed hypnosis as similar to falling in love and a female client had leaped upon him in a romantic way during hypnosis, he was startled by this event.

Due to the fact that Freud believed that psychoanalysis was superior to hypnosis, he abandoned it and developed free association. Later, in 1919, a renewed interest in hypnosis occurred when Freud mentioned blending psychoanalysis with hypnosis. In 1920, J. A. Hadfield coined the term hypnoanalysis to describe integrating hypnosis with psychoanalysis which was used to help treat shell-shocked soldiers during World War I; currently, this would be the diagnosis of posttraumatic stress disorder (PTSD). Hypnosis gained scientific respect in medicine in 1958 when the American Medical Association (AMA) accepted it as a treatment in dentistry and medicine. Finally, Division 30, Psychological Study of Hypnosis, of the American Psychological Association (APA), was founded in 1969.

SUMMARY

Clearly, hypnosis is not a new method of treatment. The Bible has several parts that describe phenomena which are hypnotic in nature. Mesmer is considered the father of modern hypnosis. Without the theoretical developments of Charcot, Janet, and others, Freud would not have been able to develop psychoanalysis. Interestingly, hypnosis and psychoanalysis continue to be isolated from the general field of psychology; however, both can explain aspects of human functioning that generally personality theories do not adequately address. Finally, hypnosis and psychoanalysis can explain many disorders such as dissociation, dissociative identity disorder, posttraumatic stress disorder (PTSD), somatoform disorder, and borderline personality disorder (Sapp 1997a,b; Sapp, Farrell, Johnson, Sartin-Kirby & Pumphrey 1997; Sapp, Ioannidis & Farrell 1995).

CLINICAL APPLICATIONS

Theories of hypnosis have direct applications to the practice of hypnosis. For example, if a clinician views hypnosis as dissociation, he or she is more likely to use techniques during hypnosis that facilitate the client's ability to experience dissociation. In contrast, clinicians viewing hypnosis as suggestions or imaginations are more likely to clinically implement suggestion strategies and guided imagery techniques. Moreover, whether hypnosis is viewed as an unconscious experience, regression, role enacting, and so forth, the conceptualization will determine the approach employed by a clinician. Finally, this is why clinicians conceptualize hypnosis differently, and this is why the practice of hypnosis is heavily linked to the history of its psychological theories.

DISCUSSION QUESTIONS

1. Because psychoanalytic theories originated from theories of hypnosis, are psychoanalytic theories necessary and sufficient to explain hypnosis?
2. What is the importance of the theory of magnetism to the development of psychological theories of hypnosis? Discuss the influences of Charcot, Janet, de Puységur, Faria, Freud, Coué, Braid, and Bernheim on the early psychological theories of hypnosis.

Chapter 3

PHENOMENA OF HYPNOSIS

APA'S DIVISION 30 DEFINITION OF HYPNOSIS

APA's Division 30 (Psychological Hypnosis) defined hypnosis, very similar to other forms of psychotherapy, as an interpersonal relationship between a client and a mental health professional in which the mental health professional offers suggestions to the client that can produce psychophysiological responses. This definition is descriptive rather than explanatory, and the phenomena of hypnosis that follow provide additional descriptions of hypnosis.

PHENOMENA OF HYPNOSIS

A definition of hypnosis is not complete without a description of its phenomena. As we discussed in Chapter 2, hypnosis is the progenitor of modern psychotherapy (Kirsch 1990). Essentially, hypnosis can be viewed as a miniature form of psychotherapy as clients' response expectancies are increased. As Sapp (1997a) demonstrated, various forms of psychotherapy differ in their effectiveness or **effect size measures.** Specifically, **meta-analyses** (statistical methods for summarizing several studies) consistently show that cognitive-behavioral treatments have the highest effect size measures (Kirsch 1990; Sapp 1997a); nevertheless, hypnosis has the largest effect size of any treatment, and it increases the effectiveness of cognitive-behavioral and dynamically oriented psychotherapies (Kirsch 1990, 1996; Kirsch, Montgomery, & Sapirstein 1995). When the effects of hypnosis match a client's expectations, treatment effectiveness increases; hence, hypnosis can change clients' expectations. To summarize, expectancy theory suggests that clients' response expectancies influence psychotherapy in general, and response expectancies are possibly one central underlying mechanism of hypnosis.

Phenomena of hypnosis include, but are not limited to, absorption, dissociation, repression, suppression, catalepsy, amnesia and hyperamnesia, analgesia and anesthesia, hyperesthesia, ideomotor and ideosensory exploration, somnambulism, hallucinations, age regression, age progression and time distortion, depersonalization, and derealization.

Absorption and Dissociation

Absorption is a client's ability to become imaginatively involved during hypnosis (Kirsch 1990). In contrast, Roche and McConkey (1990) described absorption as a trait that involves openness to cognitive and affective alterations across several situations. In addition, absorption is a client's readiness for deep mental and emotional involvement, and the client appears to be impervious to naturally distracting events. Roche and McConkey defined **imaginative involvement**, a term proposed by J. R. Hilgard (1974), as the readiness for openness to experience that involves an alteration or suspension in reality testing, and absorption involves the narrowing or expansion of consciousness.

According to Roche and McConkey (1990), absorption and imaginative involvement overlap, but they are different constructs. Plus, this researcher pointed out that absorption is a broad and complex construct that cannot be totally measured or assessed using one instrument. From this broad definition of absorption, one can conclude that absorption has trait and state dimensions; however, many clinicians and researchers assume that absorption is a relatively simple, unitary dimension (Roche & McConkey 1990). Clients who are capable of rich fantasies and very vivid imagery score highly on the Tellegen Absorption Scale (TAS), which is a standardized measure of absorption. The TAS is a 34-item (true-false but can be modified into a Likert scale) scale that measures absorption, and it correlates approximately .38 with hypnotizability (Sapp, Evanow & Arndt 1997).

Dissociation means that two or more mental processes are not integrated (Cardeña 1994). For example, dissociation is the ability to detach from one's environment such as day dreaming and seeing oneself performing actions outside of one's body. Clinically, dissociation is useful for promoting increased hypnotic depth during pain relief. In addition, it can be used to assess nonconscious processes by facilitating "automatic handwriting" for nonconscious exploration. The domain of dissociation includes normal, pathological, psychological, and neuropsychological phenomena. Some pathological phenomena include, but are not limited to, dissociative identity disorder (DID), depersonalization, derealization, dissociative amnesia, dissociative fugues, and conversion disorder (psychological factors that affect motor and sensory functioning). Neuropsychological dissociative phenomena include, but are not limited to, blindsight, commissurotomy, organic amnesia, epileptic fugues, and hemineglect.

Psychological dissociative phenomena include, but are not limited to, hypnosis, day dreaming, fantasizing, out-of-body experiences, and automatisms. Normal dissociative phenomena include, but are not limited to, self-hypnosis, fantasy proneness, and meditative fugues. During dissociation, clients' sensations, memories, and volitions may not be integrated; hence, these mental processes are dissociated. In summary, the domain of dissociation is on a continuum and it is not discrete.

The Dissociative Experiences Scale (DES) is a standardized measure of dissociation; it is a 28-item scale ranging from 0 to 100 percent. It has a test-retest reliability of .84, and it correlates with hypnotizability from .08 to .61 (Waller, Carlson & Putnam 1996). In addition, Sapp (1997c) developed the General Dissociation Scale (see Chapter 6) that allows dissociation to be assessed in the following categories based on the Diagnostic and Statistical Manual of Mental Disorders (4th Edition) (DSM-IV): dissociative identity, depersonalization, dissociative amnesia, and dissociative fugue.

Dissociative identity disorder (DID, formerly multiple personality disorder) is a client's feelings of the presence of two or more distinct personal identities within himself or herself, each with its own pattern of perceiving, relating, and thinking about the environment. **Depersonalization** is reports from clients of feeling detached from their bodies or mental processes and feeling like being in a dream world.

Dissociative amnesia is a client's inability to recall personal information such as his or her name, his or her telephone number, where he or she lives, and so forth. This inability to recall personal information is not related to alcohol or drug usage.

Dissociative fugue is where a client unexpectedly travels away from his or her home accompanied by his or her inability to recall his or her past and confusion about his or her personal identity or the presumption of a new identity.

Repression

Repression is a defense mechanism and a process through which threatening or painful thoughts, feelings, or sensations and so forth are excluded from awareness. As previously stated, repression is a process in which dissociation and other defense mechanisms can occur.

Suppression

Erdelyi (1995) showed that Sigmund Freud, not Anna Freud, used suppression and repression interchangeably. Suppression is usually a conscious attempt to avoid unwanted thoughts, feelings, sensations, and so forth. This is a conscious attempt to inhibit undesirable mental processes, and it is therefore a defense mechanism.

Catalepsy

Catalepsy is a feature of hypnosis in which a client's muscle tonicity is inhibited in such a way that limbs remain where they are positioned. Arm catalepsy is sometimes used to deepen hypnosis or to facilitate anesthesia.

Amnesia and Hyperamnesia

Changes in memory is a feature of hypnosis. **Amnesia** is the disruption or interference of memory that can be spontaneous or suggested. Hypnosis can increase the capacity of memory, called **hyperamnesia**; however, memories can be inaccurate because of suggestions from a hypnotist. In addition, memory is always a reconstructive process that is influenced by the context. It is recommended that the reader consult Chapter 6 in order to understand the complexity of hypnosis and memory.

Analgesia, Anesthesia, and Hyperesthesia

Pain has psychophysiological factors such as expectations, mental state, and so on. For susceptibility clients, hypnosis can serve as an **analgesic** to relieve pain. Seldom do clients report a total lack of pain from hypnosis. Hypnosis can serve as an **anesthesia** by reducing clients' sensitivity to pain and it can help control bleeding. Again, seldom do clients report a total insensitivity to pain as a result of hypnosis. Finally, **hyperesthesia** is when hypnosis produces an increased sensitivity to touch.

Ideomotor and Ideosensory Exploration

The **ideomotor** and **ideosensory** theory of hypnotic responding states that a therapist can communicate ideas to a client that are implanted within the client's mind and result in **automatic hypnotic responding** (ideomotor) and **automatic sensory experiences** (ideosensory). As stated in Chapter 2, James Braid used the term hypnosis, and he developed this theory of suggestion and automaticity of hypnotic responding.

Leslie LeCron and Milton Erickson independently pioneered ideomotor and ideosensory signaling or responding (Bennett 1988; LeCron 1954). The purpose of ideomotor and ideosensory signaling is to explore unconscious dynamics. Bennett (1988) presented evidence that these methods can help clients explore unconscious information that influences their behavior. Later, in Chapter 5, we will present a transcript that applies ideomotor and ideosensory responding.

Somnambulism

Somnambulism refers to a client's ability to experience one of the deepest levels of hypnosis with his or her eyes open. With clients experiencing severe pain, deep levels of hypnosis are correlated with proportional pain reduction.

Hypnotic susceptibility is the ability of a client to experience hypnosis, but susceptibility does ensure that one will experience deep levels of hypnosis. In contrast to hypnotic susceptibility, hypnotic depth is a client's subjective experience of low, medium, and deep levels of hypnosis. Clients' subjective ratings of hypnotic depth correlate significantly with objective hypnotizability measures; however, the two measures are not congruent (Sapp et al. 1997). To summarize, ideomotor and ideosensory responding is the involuntary or nonvolitional capacity of muscles and the senses to respond instantaneously to suggestions.

Hallucinations

Hallucinations are another feature of hypnosis. A negative hallucination is the client's hypnotic ability to not see or sense a stimulus that is present; whereas, a positive hallucination is a client's hypnotic capacity to experience a stimulus that is actually not present.

Hammond (1992) reported that taste, smell, and kinesthetic hallucinations are the easiest for clients to experience (36%–46% of a research sample), auditory hallucinations are the second easiest hallucinations that clients can experience (13%–17% of a research sample), and visual hallucinations are the most difficult for clients to experience (3% of a research sample).

Age Regression, Age Progression, and Time Distortion

Age regression is a client's ability to reexperience the past. Seldom do clients experience revivification or the complete reliving of the past. During regression, a client's behaviors, vocal pattern, handwriting, and so on become the way he or she believes a child would respond. Nash (1987, 1991) defined hypnosis as an adaptive form of regression in which the client returns to an earlier mode of processing information.

Very similar to age regression, **age progression** is the client's ability to fantasize or mentally rehearse situations and experiences from a future time orientation. From a diagnostic point of view, age progression can help a clinician determine how a client may react to future events of situations.

Time distortion is a client's ability to expand and to contract the subjective experiences of time. For example, 15 minutes may subjectively appear like an hour, or an hour could be perceived subjectively as 15 minutes. For the treatment of pain, time distortion can be useful for altering the sensations of pain.

Depersonalization and Derealization

Depersonalization and derealization are features of dissociation and correlates of hypnotizability. **Depersonalization** is characterized by feelings of detachment or estrangement from one's self (DSM-IV). For example, the client may feel like an automaton or as if he or she is in a dream world. **Derealization** is an alteration in a client's perception or experience of the external world, so that it seems unreal or unfamiliar.

CURRENT THEORIES OF HYPNOSIS

Even though Ericksonian hypnosis, dissociation theories, cognitive-behavioral theories, sociophenomenological theories, hypnosis as a special case of adaptive regression, and hypnosis as relaxation are the dominant theories within clinical practice, the major tension among practitioners is between the *special process* theorists and *nonstate theorists*.

Special process clinicians view hypnosis as an event or altered state of consciousness that happens to a client. Often dissociation, regression, and so on are used to explain this altered state. Some examples of altered state theories are Ericksonian practitioners, dissociation theorists, and regression theorists (Edmonston 1981; Erickson & Rossi 1979; Hilgard 1994; Nash 1987; Woody & Bowers 1994). Special process or state theorists believe that hypnosis produces trancelike, out-of-the-body, altered states of consciousness. In addition, they believe that physiologically hypnotic states differ from nonhypnotic ones.

Nonstate, social psychological, sociocognitive (social cognitive), and cognitive-behavioral practitioners do not reject the notion that drugs can produce altered states of consciousness, nor do they reject the reports from clients, during hypnosis, of changes in subjective experiences. They challenge the proposition that subjective experiences that occur during hypnosis are the consequence of an altered state of consciousness that differs from normal consciousness (Kirsch & Lynn 1998b). Kirsch and Lynn (1995) argued that one misconception of this position is that hypnotized clients are merely complying with hypnotic suggestions. These theorists view hypnotic experiences as the by-products of social experiences and cognitive-behavioral strategies used by clients. In contrast to viewing clients as passive participants, clients are viewed as the generators of hypnotic behaviors.

Ericksonian Hypnosis

Milton H. Erickson (1901-1980) founded Ericksonian hypnosis and psychotherapy and the American Society of Clinical Hypnosis (ASCH) (Erickson and Rossi 1980). He founded ASCH in 1957. There are many synonyms for Ericksonian hypnosis, such as naturalistic hypnosis, indirect hypnosis, and permissive hypnosis. From an Ericksonian perspective, hypnosis is viewed as an altered state characterized by muscle relaxation, reduced blood pressure, and a slower breathing rate. In contrast, unlike the traditional psychoanalytic view of the unconscious, Erickson viewed the unconscious as a reservoir of knowledge that can aid the client toward therapeutic change.

Traditional hypnosis is based on direct suggestions such as "you will stop smoking," "you will stop overeating," or "you must exercise." Direct suggestions are straightforward, in contrast to indirect suggestions—one hallmark of Ericksonian hypnosis—which are not direct or straightforward (Edgette & Edgette 1995). Indirect suggestions are worded in a permissive style such as "you may stop smoking" or "you can stop overeating." Here, permissive verbs such as "can" and "may" are used instead of authoritarian verbs such as "will" and "must." This moves hypnosis from a dictatorial stance toward a collaborative endeavor.

Ericksonians argue that this style of hypnosis is the most effective way to handle resistant clients and clients who score low on hypnotizability measures; however, Lynn, Neufeld, and Maré (1993) have not found any advantage to using indirect suggestions. And Sapp (1997b) did not find statistical significant differences between indirect and direct hypnosis.

ture which contains cognitions, affects, and memories. Moreover, Ericksonian therapists emphasize the client's internal resources and inherent capacities for change. Another feature of Ericksonian hypnosis is tailoring hypnosis to the individual needs of the client, and many Ericksonian therapists believe that hypnotizability is directly proportional to the degree that hypnosis is tailored to the client (Edgette & Edgette 1995).

Yet another feature of Ericksonian hypnosis is multilevel communication (attempting to communicate with the client through several modes of communication). For example, indirect suggestion, often through metaphors, stories, poems, and aphorisms are features of multilevel communication. Erickson was also known for paradoxical intention, pacing and leading; often, he would make suggestions that matched his clients' overt behaviors. First, Erickson would pace his clients, matching clients' nonverbal behaviors. Next, he would lead which is the more direct aspect of Ericksonian hypnosis. To summarize, even though Ericksonian hypnosis is characterized by indirect suggestions, Erickson would often give his clients directives or direct suggestions. In Chapter 5, we will provide a transcript for an Ericksonian induction.

Zeig and Rennick (1991) pointed out that the Ericksonian approach is a **communications model to hypnosis**, where formal trance or inductions may or may not be employed. What is important is the interpersonal communication with the client that taps unconscious capacities. Haley (1967, 1973) noted that Erickson was one of the first generation of brief strategic psychotherapists. Whereas Haley described the interpersonal aspects of Ericksonian hypnosis, Ernest Rossi (Erickson & Rossi 1979, 1981, 1989) elucidated forms of indirect suggestions, the utilization approach, and intrapsychic dimensions of Erickson's approach.

Bandler and Grinder (1975) and Grinder, Delozier, and Bandler (1977) focused on the communications aspects of Ericksonian psychotherapy by developing neurolinguistic programming (NLP). They emphasized the transformational grammar and sensory-based elements of perceptions and representations. Representations or representation systems deal with the patterns clients use in storing information such as seeing, hearing, and feeling. The two major techniques utilized by NLP are anchoring and reframing.

Anchoring is the process by which a therapist focuses on changing a client's undesirable emotional states by targeting specific stimuli such as touch, sound, facial expressions, and postural changes. The purpose of anchoring is to evoke new feelings within the client. **Reframing** is the process of getting the client to interpret his or her behavior from different perspectives.

The claims that Bandler and Grinder (1975) made about NLP, such as curing phobias in less than an hour; helping children and adults with learning disabilities in less than an hour; eliminating habit disorders, such as smoking, drinking, and overeating, in a few sessions has not held up to research investigations (Coe & Scharcoff 1985; Dowd & Hingst 1983; Dowd & Petty 1982; Gumm, Walker & Day 1982; Henry 1984). In addition, research has not substantiated that clients make mental maps of the world by processing sensory information through auditory, visual, and kinesthetic input. NLP hypothesizes that clients prefer certain primary representational systems (e.g., visual).

During the 1980s, many practitioners moved away from NLP and embraced Ericksonian approaches to hypnosis because research (McConkey 1984, 1986; Van Gorp, Myer & Dunbar 1985) did not find NLP to live up to its claims and that NLP was not found to be superior to hypnosis. Finally, in terms of suggestions for analgesia, experimental evidence suggests that direct suggestions are more effective than indirect suggestions (Van Gorp et al. 1985).

Dissociation Theories

As stated in Chapter 2, Charcot and his student, Janet, popularized the dissociation theory of hypnosis. They hypothesized that dissociation was more likely if a client had a predisposition to a weak nervous system or was traumatized. This theory stated hypnosis resulted in dissociation, the separation of clients' ideations.

Hilgard (1994) modified Janet's theory of hypnosis into what he called **neodissociation**. Hilgard's theory is an incomplete theory of dissociation based on information processing. Essentially, Hilgard stated that cognitive subsystems or structures that are arranged in a hierarchy can become separated (dissociated) from the executive ego, processing can occur outside of one's level of awareness (unconscious), and information can become available on another level (conscious). This is what is meant by divided consciousness, the dissociation of unconscious from conscious material.

The **neodissociation theory** states that hypnotic responding is involuntary and nonvolitional. To say that hypnotic responding is nonvolitional suggests that hypnotic experiences appear to happen automatically. At the least, this is the subjective experience some clients report. Moreover, nonvolitional suggests that clients' experiences occur without conscious volitional effort. Furthermore, the term involuntary has the connotation of being unpreventable and occurring against the client's will (Kirsch 1990). Even though hypnotically responsive clients report their experiences as occurring without their direct volitional effort, they are aware that they could terminate responding at any point (Kirsch 1990). Hilgard stated that a combination of dissociation and an amnesic barrier among dissociated subsystems explains why clients experience hypnosis as involuntary and nonvolitional.

To summarize, the neodissociation theory of hypnosis states that behavior is arranged as a hierarchical series of subsystems that produce habitual actions and sequences. The executive ego controls the inputs and outputs of the subsystems; however, once cognitive subsystems are activated, they can carry out habital actions with limited involvement of executive ego. For example, when one is able to arrive at a habitual destination (one's home), without remembering the cognitive process and action sequences (Kirsch & Lynn 1998a,b).

The major difficulty this writer has with Hilgard's (1991) neodissociation theory is the following quote from Hilgard: "Hypnosis enters because effective suggestions from the hypnotist take much of the normal control away from the subject. That is, the hypnotist may influence the executive functions themselves and change the hierarchical arrangements of the substructures" (p. 98). The previous quote suggests that the client gives control to the hypnotist; however, this writer questions how and why a client would need to relinquish even partial control during a process that is self-induced, self-hypnosis. This writer does not question how Hilgard explains dissociation, especially for pain control, but Hilgard's notion of an amnesic-barrier is unnecessary to explain dissociation and involuntary hypnotic responding. Moreover, this writer believes that Kirsch and Lynn's (1998a,b) new social-cognitive theory of dissociation offers a more general explanation of hypnotic involuntariness; however, this writer also critiques Kirsch and Lynn's new theory in Chapter 6. Finally, the theory that follows, Woody and Bowers (1994), also questions Hilgard's theory of an amnesic-barrier.

Woody and Bowers (1994) presented a **dissociated control theory of hypnosis**. They stated that hypnosis did not involve the division, separation, or dissociation of consciousness, but the dissociation of cognitive and behavior subsystems from the executive ego's control; hence, systems are activated by lower level functions. From this perspective, dissociation is the result of frontal lobe dysfunction or inhibition. Similarly to Hilgard's theory, the dissociated control theory of hypnosis views hypnosis as an involuntary and nonvolitional process and an altered state of consciousness. Nevertheless, the dissociated control theory questions Hilgard's theory of the division of the executive ego into conscious and unconscious parts that are separated by an amnesic barrier.

The **dissociated control theory** posits that dissociation mimics **frontal lobe disorders**; hence, frontal lobe dysfunction is brought about through hypnosis and an altered state of consciousness. Nevertheless, neuro-imaging techniques have not located physiological substrates of hypnotic responding. More specifically, constructs that correspond to a hypnotic trance have not been located from physiological research. What has been obtained from physiological research is why some clients respond to certain suggestions, but a distinct state of hypnosis has not been located from the physiological research.

Currently, a major issue of the dissociation theories is how much does hypnotic responding differ as a result of **attentional resources**? For example, clinically, one would assume that clients with inattentive disorders would not be very hypnotizable, due to the fact that they have difficulty attending to hypnotic suggestions; in fact, Barabasz and Barabasz (1996) found that clients with attention deficit hyperactivity disorder were extremely hypnotizable. Moreover, in 1999, Mr. James T. Kirsch, one of the author's students conducting research on hypnosis and inattention, found that college students with extreme scores on inattention measures were very hypnotizable.

Actually, Kirsch, Burgess, and Braffman (1999) predicted, according to the dissociated control theory, that hypnotic responding should not require attentional effort, and hypnotic responses should not be impeded or affected by cognitive load. In contrast, the neodissociation theory would predict that cognitive load would impede responses to hypnotic suggestions. Kirsch et al. found that attentional resources were required for memory recall and memory suppression; however, their research also suggests that various hypnotic suggestions such as challenge, ideomotor, and subjective experiences may require variable attentional resources. Specifically, they found that cognitive load inhibited the subjective experience for challenge suggestions, but cognitive load did not inhibit the behavioral expressions of challenge suggestions. It appears that subjective experiences elicited by challenge suggestions require attentional effort or resources. Finally, apparently attentional resources are required to initiate suggested subjective experiences, and attentional effort is needed for memory recall and memory suppression.

Cognitive-Behavioral Theories

Cognitive-behavioral theories of hypnosis are referred to as **sociocognitive** and **social psychological**, and they are **nonstate**

approaches to hypnosis. There are two common misconceptions of the cognitive-behavioral camp. First, it does not deny the reality and significance of hypnotic phenomena; second, it does not question clients' abilities to alter their subjective experiences during hypnosis (Kirsch 1993). What cognitive-behavioral theorists question is the importance of the concept hypnotic trance in explaining clients' experiences.

Specifically, Barber (1969), Sarbin and Coe (1972), and Spanos (1986) rejected explicitly the hypnotic trance or state theory of hypnosis. Barber viewed hypnosis as goal-directed behavior; Spanos viewed hypnosis as clients' abilities to use cognitive-behavioral strategies and other goal-directed behaviors; and Kirsch (1990), taking a social learning point of view, posited that hypnosis is the result of clients' expectations. Furthermore, Sarbin and Coe used "role enactment" theory, a social psychological construct, to explain hypnosis.

Five points substantiate the cognitive-behavioral perspectives of hypnosis. **First**, there are not any consistent physiological markers of hypnosis. Even though physiological data are beginning to show why certain clients respond differently to suggestions, hypothesized hypnotic states have not been found (Kirsch & Lynn 1998b; Sarbin & Slagle 1979). **Second**, hypnotic phenomena can be produced without hypnotic inductions (Barber 1969). Barber found that hypnotic inductions were not necessary to elicit hypnosis and that clients' expectations and motivations could produce hypnotic phenomena.

Third, hypnotic inductions produce a small increase in suggestibility. In addition, other techniques such as guided imagery, meditation, and placebo pills can duplicate or surpass the effects of a hypnotic induction (Glass & Barber 1961; Katz 1979; Vickery, Kirsch, Council & Sirkin 1985; Sapp, Farrell, Johnson, Sartin-Kirby & Pumphrey 1996). Sarbin and Coe (1972) argued that when clients enact their roles of how they think hypnotized clients are supposed to respond, the result is hypnotic phenomena.

Fourth, McConkey (1984, 1986) found that clients described their hypnotic experiences as a "normal" state of focused attention (absorption) and imaginative involvement. Moreover, McConkey did not find that the majority of clients reported their hypnotic experiences as altered states of consciousness. **Lastly**, the descriptions clients give about progressive relaxation training do not markedly differ from ones to standard hypnotic inductions (Kirsch, Mobayed, Council & Kenny 1992; Sapp 1995).

Clearly, cognitive-behavioral theorists take a nonstate view of hypnosis that challenges the trance-like, out-of-body, and altered state of consciousness theories. In addition, these theorists do not believe that hypnotized clients are merely complying with suggestions; in contrast, they view clients as using social influences and cognitive-behavioral strategies to produce hypnosis. Neither do these theorists question the domain of dissociation.

Sociophenomenological Theories

Shor (1959), Tellegen and Atkinson (1974), Orne (1979), and Laurence and Perry (1983) stated that hypnosis is the result of goal-directed behaviors (cognitive-behavioral strategies) and an altered state of consciousness. These theorists researched the experiential and cognitive style correlates of hypnosis, and they incorporate ideas from both the special process and nonstate positions. These theories place an emphasis on the interactive nature of multiple variables during hypnosis and at times are referred to as "interactive-phenomenological theories." Furthermore, clients' personality traits and abilities tend to shape the methods of studying hypnotic experiences. In fact, members of this theoretical approach tend to examine the interrelationship among personality, cognitive, social-psychological factors, and hypnosis with clients. This approach attempts to capture the multidimensional nature of hypnosis.

Psychological Regression

Nash (1987, 1991) viewed hypnosis as a **special case of adaptive psychological regression**, and his theory is a psychodynamic one. Gruenewald, Fromm, and Oberlander (1979) defined adaptive regression as the global return to earlier modes of processing information; this is a shift from "higher" mental processes to "lower" ones.

Schilder (1956) was the progenitor to viewing hypnosis as adaptive regression. Schilder stated that only part of the ego becomes involved during hypnosis, and a part of the ego maintains contact with the external world. However, pathological regression is the total paralysis or helplessness of the ego. Many of the ego's functions during hypnosis occur through the client's transference relationship with his or her therapist who professionally elicits hypnosis. Very similar to the dissociation theories, this theoretical position conceptualizes hypnosis as a trance and an altered state of consciousness. To illustrate, the greater the degree of hypnotic trance, the greater the client's ego functions are moderated through his or her therapist.

Gill and Brenman (1959) stated explicitly that the client's ego controls hypnotic regression. During hypnosis, they believed that as opposed to regression occurring in the entire ego, a portion or subsystem of the client's ego regresses and searches for derivatives of a regressed state. One important point about this process is that the ego does not lose contact with reality.

It was Nash (1991) who found that adaptive regression is not congruent to earlier stages of human development. He argued that hypnosis is not temporal regression or revivification, a complete reliving of the past, but topographic regression, or a reversal in space but not time.

Nash stated that hypnosis is a condition in which subsystems of the ego experiences topographical regression that produce changes in the self and others. For example, some of these changes include shifts from secondary processing to primary processing, increased affect, increased transference relationship with the therapist, changes in bodily experiences, and alterations in volition. To summarize, Nash stated that topographical regression is the primary determining feature of hypnosis in which transference phenomena represents one of many potential shifts in ego functioning. Finally, Nash viewed hypnosis as shifts in the ways clients process information.

From a clinical perspective, one major implication of Nash's work is that hypnotic regression does not involve clients returning to earlier developmental stages of functioning. When Nash tested clients who returned to earlier childhood levels of intellectual functioning, he found that hypnotically-regressed clients' intellectual functioning was comparable to that of normal adults. Specifically, hypnotically-regressed clients were not more childlike than nonhypnotized clients who role-played as hypnotic controls. Nash's research shows that hypnotically-regressed clients' intellectual functioning is that of adults and not children. Finally, using a **psychodynamic orientation**, Nash stated that hypnosis is a special case of adaptive psychological regression. His position is similar to that of dissociation theories in that he maintains that hypnosis is an altered state of consciousness.

Relaxation Theory of Hypnosis

Edmonston (1981, 1991) presented a single factor theory of hypnosis called **anesis**, which comes from the Greek and means "to relax or let go." This is a single-factor theory of hypnosis that states that anesis or relaxation precedes all hypnotic phenomena. In fact, anesis is a two-step process. First, the client receives relaxation, followed by changes in alertness and suggestions by a clinician. And characteristics of anesis include hypersuggesibility, spontaneous amnesia, and the subjective experience of involuntariness. According to Edmonston, anesis enhances disinhibition, attitudes, motivation, ego functioning, dissociation, and role playing with clients.

Edmonston found when he compared clients who had received traditional hypnotic inductions and relaxation inductions that clients' responses on electrodermal responses such as conditioning, heart rate, and oral temperature were the same. This suggested that hypnosis and relaxation share much of the same physiology. Furthermore, Edmonston found that hypnosis and nonhypnotic relaxation were equally effective in reducing tension, stress, and anxiety with clients.

In addition, Edmonston sees similarities between behavior therapies and hypnosis. Even when he compared hypnosis with nonhypnotic relaxation to treat hypertension, migraine headaches, insomnia, and anxiety, the findings were the same: nonhypnotic relaxation produces results that are equivalent to hypnosis.

Interestingly, Sapp (1997) describes two kinds of relaxation—cognitive and motoric; however, Edmonston views both as part of the same process, and he believes that the two processes are inseparable. In terms of alert hypnosis and anesis, Edmonston views them as differing in kind rather than degree. And he views alert hypnosis as relaxation produced through an active process in contrast to a passive one.

Finally, Edmonston believes that relaxation can produce differences in cognition, primary process mentation, dissociation, regression, and other phenomena associated with hypnosis. He stated that it was anesis or relaxation, not dissociation, regression, role enactment, cognitive behavioral strategies, or expectations, that form the fundamental basis of hypnosis. Finally, he viewed dissociation, role enactment, psychological regression, and so on as by-products of anesis or relaxation; and he saw relaxation as the mechanism of hypnosis.

CLINICAL APPLICATIONS

Regression, cognitive-behavioral, dissociation, relaxation, and absorption features of hypnosis are useful for clinical practice. For example, clients experiencing severe pain often benefit from relaxation, dissociation, and cognitive-behavioral strategies. In addition, dissociation and regression aspects of hypnosis give clinicians the potential to treat a variety of related disorders such as dissociated identity disorder (DID), borderline personality disorder, somatoform disorder, and posttraumatic stress disorder (PTSD), all of which have dissociation as a major feature. In

Chapter 5, we will provide a variety of transcripts that can be applied to these overlapping dissociative disorders.

DISCUSSION QUESTIONS

1. What are the clinical implications of viewing hypnosis as an altered state of consciousness?
2. From a clinical standpoint, how important is it that hypnotic responsiveness can be modifiable?
3. For the treatment of pain, which theory or group of theories offer the most applications?
4. Even though APA's definition of hypnosis is only descriptive, describe the phenomena of hypnosis.
5. What is the contention between special process and nonstate theorists?

Chapter 4

DISSOCIATIVE DISORDERS

THE DIAGNOSTIC AND STATISTICAL MANUAL OF MENTAL DISORDERS (DSM-IV) defined **dissociative disorders** as disruptions in consciousness, memory, sense of identity, or the perceptions of one's environment. These disorders overlap with acute stress disorder, posttraumatic stress disorder (PTSD), and somatoform disorders.

Acute stress disorder and **PTSD** are anxiety disorders. Specifically, a client meets the diagnosis of acute stress disorder when he or she experiences anxiety, and dissociative symptoms within one month of being exposed to an extreme or traumatic stressor. The DSM-IV criteria requires that the client, either while experiencing the traumatic event or afterward, have a minimum of three of the following dissociative symptoms: a phenomenological or subjective sense of numbing, detachment (absence of emotional responsiveness), the reduction in the awareness of one's environment, derealization, depersonalization, or dissociative amnesia. After the trauma, the traumatic event is reexperienced as dreams, images, illusions, flashbacks, and so on. The client attempts to avoid people, places, and things that produce recollections of the trauma. Another feature of this disorder is the client has difficulty sleeping, concentrating, and experiences of extreme anxiety, exaggerated startle response, and motor restlessness. The symptoms of acute stress disorder significantly interfere with social, occupational, and other areas of functioning. This anxiety disorder lasts at least two days and does not extend beyond four weeks of the traumatic event. Finally, the symptoms are not due to the effects of drugs, medications, or a general medical condition.

Clients with acute stress disorder, as a result of a traumatic event, develop dissociative symptoms, and they find it difficult if not impossible to experience pleasure. The specific dissociative experiences are feeling detached from one's body, experiencing the world as surreal, difficulty concentrating, and difficulty recalling specific aspects of the event (dissociative amnesia). Some associated features of this disorder are feelings of despair, feelings of hopelessness, and major depression. If the symptoms of acute stress disorder persist for more than a month, a client is diagnosed with PTSD.

Somatoform disorders are the presence of physical symptoms that mimic a medical condition; however, these physical symptoms cannot be explained by general medical conditions or by other psychological disorders such as anxiety disorders. The DSM-IV defines the following somatoform disorders: somatization disorder, undifferentiated somatoform disorder, conversion disorder, pain disorder, hypochondriasis, body dysmorphic disorder, and somatoform disorder not otherwise specified.

Historically, called **hysteria** or **Briquet's syndrome**, somatization disorder is a polysymptomatic disorder that begins before the age of 30. It is characterized by pain, gastrointestinal, sexual, and pseudoneurological symptoms.

Undifferentiated somatoform disorder is characterized by physical symptoms that last at least six months, but these symptoms do not warrant the diagnosis of somatization disorder because they are below the threshold of a somatization disorder.

Conversion disorder is the presence of unexplained symptoms that suggest a neuropsychological condition; however, psychological factors account for the physical symptoms. A diagnosis of conversion disorder is not made if it is discovered that a client is malingering or feigning symptoms. When psychological factors play a significant role in the onset, severity, exacerbation, and continuation of pain, this characterizes a pain disorder. A **pain disorder** can be associated with psychological and medical conditions. Partly, because 10 percent to 15 percent of adults in the United States experience work disability connected with back pain, pain disorder is relatively common.

Hypochondriasis is the preoccupation and fear of having a serious disease based on the client's misinterpretation of bodily symptoms. Often, the client has poor insight in that he or she does not recognize that his or her concern about having a serious illness is excessive. The prevalence of this disorder within general medical practice has been reported between 4 percent and 9 percent.

Body dysmorphic disorder, historically known as dysmorphobia, is the excessive preoccupation with defects in one's appearance. If excessive preoccupation is restricted to fatness, a diagnosis of body dysmorphic disorder is not made and the clinician should consider a diagnosis of anorexia nervosa. Moreover, if the client's preoccupation is restricted to discomfort about his or her primary and secondary sex characteristic, a possible diagnosis of gender identity disorder may be in order. The reader may want to consult the DSM-IV for possible differential diagnoses associated with body dysmorphic disorder.

Lastly, **somatoform disorder not otherwise specified** include disorders with somatoform symptoms that do not meet the exact criteria of specific somatoform disorders. Pseudocyesis, a false belief of being pregnant, is one example of this category of disorder. Accompanying symptoms of pseudocyesis are an enlarged abdomen, reduced menstrual flow, subjective feelings of fetal movements, amenorrhea, nausea, mamillary gland engorgement and secretions, and labor pains during the expected date of delivery. What is interesting about this disorder is that endocrine changes can be present, but they cannot be explained by general medical conditions.

BORDERLINE PERSONALITY DISORDER

The United States, Canada, Mexico, Israel, Sweden, Denmark, and Russia have found **borderline personality disorders** within their populations (Kreisman & Straus 1989). These writers suggest that personalities such as Marilyn Monroe, Saddam Hussein, Moamar Kadafi, Adolf Hitler, and others were borderline personalities. Some clinicians such as Loranger, Oldham, and Tulis (1982); Baron (1985); and Gunderson (1984) consider dissociative identity disorder (DID) as a special case of borderline personality disorder (BPD). Fyer (1988) found a high percentage (up to 82% of clients) of BPD in clients with DID. Nace, Saxon, and Shore (1983) found a high incidence of BPD in clients diagnosed with PTSD. Moreover, BPD overlaps with other personality disorders such as dependent and avoidant.

BPD has been compared to schizophrenia and affective disorders. Schizophrenics tend to be comfortable with hallucinations and delusion, while BPD clients can be disturbed by their perceptual distortions. Additionally, BPD clients are not as severely disturbed as schizophrenic clients, and BPD clients are not as impaired socially (Kreisman & Straus, 1989). BPD clients can have mood swings that are similar to bipolar (manic-depressive) disorder; however, BPD clients' moods tend to be more unpredictable and transient than clients with affective disorders. Finally, the diagnoses anorexia nervosa and bulimia are associated with BPD. The extremes (absolutistic thinking) that anorexics have of seeing themselves as totally fat or totally thin and employing binging and purging are a means to maintain the distorted illusion of self-control.

In 1938, Adolph Stern coined the term "borderline" to describe clients who were not neurotic or psychotic but somewhere between the two classifications. Often, projective tests and other unstructured assessments bring out the regressed and childlike thinking of BPD clients. Obviously, some clinicians view BPD as prepsychotic or as latent schizophrenia.

Specifically, the DSM-IV defined BPD as a pervasive pattern of unstableness within interpersonal relationships, self-image, affect and marked impulsivity starting in early adulthood. A diagnosis of BPD can be made if the presence of five or more of the following exists with a client:

1. Frantic attempts to avoid real or imagined feelings of abandonment.

2. Patterns of unstable and intense relationships that range between idealized love and devaluations in terms of hate. Often these clients vacillate between extreme love and extreme hate.

3. Unstable self-image characterized by marked and persistent identity disturbances.

4. Impulsivity in at least two self-damaging areas such as overspending, promiscuous sex, substance abuse, reckless driving, and binge eating.

5. Recurring suicidal behaviors such as threats of suicide and self-mutilation, especially cutting oneself.

6. Marked swings in mood that usually last a few hours and seldom more than a few days.

7. Persistent feelings of emptiness.

8. Anger management difficulty. This can involve difficulty controlling anger, such as frequent outbursts of anger, constant anger, and physically acting out.

9. Stress-related paranoid ideations or transient or severe dissociative symptoms.

To summarize, individuals with BPD attempt frantically to avoid real or imagined abandonment or separation. The client's self-image is based upon psychological fusing with others. When a client gets the perception that he or she will be abandoned, he or she will respond with intense anger, and the client will have intense feelings of fear and despair.

During initial periods of relationships, BPD clients will attempt to become enmeshed with the person he or she is in a relationship with. Initially, the client will idealize his or her partner or friend; later, within the relationship, the client will devalue his or her friend or partner. Clients with this disorder may have issues with their self-image and will often wonder if they exist. The client's self-image is based on extremes such as "good" or "bad" or "right" or "wrong." It is not uncommon for clients to have changes in their self-image characterized by drastic changes in career, values, vocational aspirations, and gender identity.

Impulsivity is another feature of this disorder. For example, clients with this disorder will often spend money irresponsibly, gamble, drive recklessly, binge eat, abuse substances, and engage in unsafe sex.

Suicidal gestures are another feature of this disorder. For example, recurrent suicidal behavior, threats, gestures, and self-mutilation are part of this syndrome. The DSM-IV reported that completed suicide occurs in 8 percent to 10 percent of these clients. And self-mutilation often occurs in the form of cutting and burning.

There are many associated features of this disorder. Many clients will undermine themselves at the moment that their goals will be realized. For example, dropping out of college just before graduation or destroying a good relationship when it is clear it can last. Hallucinations, body-image distortions, and hypnagogic phenomena can occur as well as other psychotic-like symptoms. Inanimate or transitional objects can mean more to a client's sense of security than interpersonal relationships. For example, a pet or a teddy bear can serve as objects of security. When BPD clients have mood disorders and substance-related disorders, suicide is more likely to occur. Physical abuse, sexual abuse, neglect, and parental loss are commonly reported in these clients' childhood histories.

Interestingly, BPD is diagnosed mostly in females, and the DSM-IV reports that it is seen in cultures around the world. It is estimated that about 2 percent of the general population experience BPD, about 10 percent of outpatient mental health clinic patients experience BPD, and 20 percent of inpatient psychiatric patients experience BPD. Between 30 percent and 60 percent of populations experiencing a personality disorder also experience BPD. In terms of familial patterns, BPD does run within families, and it is five times more likely among first-degree biological relatives (DSM-IV). Finally, BPD can coexist with mood disorders and other personality disorders. In conclusion, instability of self-image, interpersonal relationships, and affect are characteristics of BPD. The next section discusses hypnosis applications.

HYPNOSIS APPLICATIONS FOR BPD

Caution should be exercises when considering to use hypnosis with the BPD client. A recurrent theme of this text is that a therapist should only use hypnosis for psychological disorders in which he or she has specialized training; however, if one has the requisite training, many general hypnotic techniques can be employed such as ego-strengthening, regression, anxiety and stress reduction, and so on. The reader can consult Chapter 5 for a variety of hypnosis treatment transcripts. In addition, maintaining distinct psychological boundaries can be difficult with the BPD client; therefore an understanding of the theories of Fromm and Nash (see Chapter 5) and other psychoanalytic theorists can be useful. Moreover, hypnosis can be used to help clients maintain constant rather than fragmented self-object representation.

From a therapeutic process point of view, the therapist must provide a safe environment where the BPD client can recapitulate the development of the separation-individuation period. Many of the object-relations, theorists, psychodynamic schools of thought, view BPD as caused by a client having difficulties during the differentiation and separation/individuation processes. Essentially, object-relations theorists elucidate the process a client undergoes to become an individual. Here, the object refers to significant persons from the client's past (Fromm & Nash 1997; Sapp 1997). To reiterate, hypnosis can help a client to develop object constancy and learn how to establish and maintain boundaries. Finally, self-hypnosis can provide the BPD client with a technique that helps him or her self-regulate the symptoms of BPD.

OVERVIEW OF DISSOCIATIVE IDENTITY DISORDER (DID)

Kluft (1991) noted that diagnoses of **DID** are increasing in frequency, and this dissociative disorder is of considerable interest to clinicians who work with dissociative disorders and who are familiar with clinical hypnosis. DID is a controversial entity. This is due to the fact that dissociation is a complex construct, and DID is closely correlated with reported histories of child abuse; nevertheless, not all abused children develop a dissociative disorder. Therefore, probably, there is not a causal relationship between DID and reported histories of child abuse. Clinicians who are uncomfortable with child abuse use denial and derealization to distort clients' accounts of abuse. Often, this leads to clinicians who experience countertransference toward DID clients, and these feelings can be overwhelming and clinicians defend against such emotions by disavowing the credibility of clients' accounts. Within the older literature, iatrogenesis was connected with DID when hypnosis was cited as the treatment (Kluft, 1991), and Kluft (1982, 1991) argued that such reports are artifacts.

Description of DID

DID is a dissociative disorder that involves disturbances in memory and identity. What distinguishes DID from other dissociative disorders is the presence of two or more distinct personalities within a client. Essentially, the awareness among or between personalities can exist on a continuum where awareness of the various personalities can vary dramatically. Specifically, patterns of amnesia can be minimal, partial, or complete; therefore, amnesia can exist along a continuum.

Clients with DID may display PTSD symptoms such as flashbacks and startle responses. In addition, these clients can self-mutilate and make suicidal and aggressive gestures. Some clients continue repetitive relationships with other individuals that involve physical and sexual abuse. For example, if a female was abused as a child by a relative, it is not unlikely that she will continue a stormy relationship with that adult into adulthood. The preceding description of DID parallels some of the features of borderline personality disorder.

In terms of research findings, clients with DID tend to score toward the upper range on hypnotizability and dissociation scales (see Chapter 6). There can be variations in physiological functioning across identity states. For example, personalities may show differences in handwriting, differences in visual acuity, a difference in pain tolerance, and so on.

Specifically, DSM-IV criteria for DID are as follows:

1. A client with two or more distinct personalities. Each personality has its unique way of relating, thinking, and perceiving the self and the environment.

2. Two or more identities or personality states recurrently take control of the client's behavior.

3. The lack of ability to recall important personal information. The symptoms of DID cannot be due to blackouts that result from substance abuse or from a general medical condition, such as seizures. With children, symptoms of DID cannot be attributed to imaginary playmates or fantasy.

Clients with DID have difficulty acknowledging amnesia. Some clients equate amnesia with psychosis, and other clients get accustomed to dissociation of time, and they assume that their amnesia is normal. Personalities can be aware of varying aspects of each other. For example, they may experience each other as friends, relatives, adversaries, and so on. Even though some personalities may be aware of others, there may not be direct interaction with them.

In terms of gender differences, DID is diagnosed three to nine times more often in adult women than in adult men. Females tend to average 15 or more identities. In contrast, males average about 8 identities. Paralleling patterns of BPD, DID clients may show fewer symptoms as they get into their forties; however, psychosocial stressors and substance abuse can cause symptoms to reemerge.

Some clinicians believe that male clients with DID experience difficulty with the criminal justice system, and they end up in jail rather than the mental health system.

Differential Diagnosis and DID

Axis I and Axis II diagnoses can coexist with DID without explaining it (Benner & Joscelyne, 1984; Coryell, 1983; Kluft, 1991). Clary, Burstin, and Carpenter (1984) discuss DID as a borderline personality and narcissistic variant. Horevitz and Braun (1984) found that 70 percent of DID clients also met the diagnosis of borderline personality disorder. In contrast to viewing DID as a variant of a personality disorder, Kluft (1991) concluded that DID and personality disorder are distinct disorders; however, they can coexist within the same client.

Fink (1991) found that personality disorders (Axis II diagnoses) can coexist with DID globally within an individual, or they can be found within an alter. Kluft (1991) reported that 90 percent of DID clients also meet the diagnosis of depression. In addition, it is not uncommon for dissociative episodes to occur within depression.

Many DID clients were once diagnosed as schizophrenic. This is due to the hallucinations or alters' voice, the presence of alters, and the sense of delusion experienced by the core personality and sometimes by alters' overlap with symptoms of schizophrenia. In terms of hallucinations, many schizophrenics report that hallucinations occur outside their heads; in contrast, DID clients often report that hallucinations occur within their heads. In addition, DID clients are able to reality test once they are stabilized, and they can maintain good rapport with their therapists.

When a client is charged with a legal violation, malingering is a possible differential diagnosis. Kluft (1991) argued that when clients overstate their cases and do not maintain the consistency of their alters, malingering may be occurring. Finally, malingering is a complicated issue with DID clients because a number of these clients commit antisocial acts that are illegal; therefore, it is possible for a DID client whose alter has committed a crime to malinger.

Treatment of DID

Even though there is some controversy in the treatment of DID, many experienced clinicians attempt to **integrate personalities**. In addition, many clinicians experienced with DID clients tend to use hypnosis as a treatment to associate or assimilate alters. Like the treatment of clients with borderline personality, DID clients need prolonged and intense treatment. Treatment involves getting the personalities to work toward the goal of unification, integration, or fusion.

Wilbur (1986) and Kluft (1991) found that a minority of clients with DID who have ego strength can undergo psychoanalysis and forego hypnosis; however, Kluft recommends combining psychoanalytic psychotherapy with hypnosis for the majority of DID clients.

The International Society for the Study of Dissociation (ISSD) has developed treatment guidelines for the treatment of dissociative disorders. Also, Kluft (1991), Putnam (1994), and Ross (1989) have provided a general outline for treatment.

The **first step** in terms of successful treatment is the establishment of a therapeutic alliance with the presenting personality and individually with each alternate personality (alter).

The **second phase** of treatment is making a diagnosis. Putnam, Guroff, Silberman, Barban, and Post (1986) listed the following as indices of DID:

1. Previous treatment failures.
2. Several previous diagnoses.
3. Concurrent psychophysiological (somatic) symptoms.
4. Disorientation and distortions of time.
5. Lapses in one's perception of time.
6. Family members and friends noting changes in one's behavior.
7. Discovering possessions and changes in one's handwriting that cannot be accounted for or recognized.
8. Hearing voices within one's head.
9. The corroboration of a history of child abuse.

10. Amnesia for childhood events from the ages of six to eleven.
11. Using "we" in a collective sense.
12. Severe headaches.
13. The elicitation of alternate personalities through Amytal or hypnosis.

Whalen and Nash (1996) provided a thorough discussion about the relationship between hypnosis and dissociation. They argued that there is no compelling evidence to support the proposition that hypnotizability and dissociation are overlapping traits. Within clinical samples, the correlation between hypnotizability and dissociation range from .08, $p > .05$ to .17, $p > .05$. For nonclinical samples, correlations range from .11, $p > .05$ to .20, $p < .05$.

Sapp and Evanow (1998) found that the Creative Imagination Scale (CIS), an imaginative measure of hypnosis, correlated .21 with dissociation, $p < .05$ for college students. In addition, the Harvard Group Scale of Hypnotic Susceptibility, Form A (HGSHS:A) correlated .19 with dissociation, $p < .05$.
Likewise, Sapp and Evanow found that the CIS correlated significantly with absorption, $r = .43$, $p < .05$, and the HGSHS:A also correlated significantly with absorption, $r = .36$, $p < .05$. It is clear that hypnotizability, dissociation, and absorption are correlated; however, the correlations are often low and nonsignificant. Clearly, these constructs are not synonymous personality structures (Faith & Ray 1994).

Some clinicians assume that trauma such as child abuse causes severe dissociation or dissociative disorders. Nash, Lynn, and Givens (1984) did find that hypnotizability was correlated with abuse that occurred in childhood. These researchers reported a correlation between hypnotizability and reports of childhood abuse of .30. Whalen and Nash (1996) reported that the correlation between trauma and dissociation ranges from .25 to .45. One difficulty with these findings is that operational definitions of trauma cause methodological difficulties in the literature. For example, many researchers and theorists assume that any physical or sexual abuse is traumatic; nevertheless, every abused child will not develop traumatic symptoms.

The area of dissociation, like trauma research, is not without methodological difficulties. The Dissociative Experiences Scale (DES) is the most widely used measure of dissociation. Even though the DES has acceptable psychometric properties, Nash, Hulsey, Sexton, Harralson, and Lambert (1993) found that high scores in the DES can be attributable to gross psychopathology and not dissociative pathology. Sapp developed the General Dissociation Scale, a new dissociation scale based on DSM-IV criteria, to assess dissociative disorders (see Chapter 6).

To summarize, evidence suggests that trauma and dissociation are linked, but Nash et al. (1993) questioned if this link is linear, and second, they question if this link forms a cause-effect relationship. The relationships among hypnosis, dissociation, and trauma appear complex and indirect. In addition, there is not a developmental pathway that explains how these three constructs can coexist. Perhaps longitudinal studies within the area of developmental psychology will provide definitive quantitative data on the possible causal pathways that could link hypnosis, dissociation, and trauma. Finally, even though a therapist may have clinical reasons for using hypnosis to treat DID, definitive research that investigates the utility of hypnosis in treating DID is needed.

The **third** phase of treatment is establishing communication with the accessible alters. This phase assumes that the client was screened for DID by such items of the Dissociative Experience Scale (DES) (Bernstein and Putnam 1986) or the General Dissociation Scale (see Chapter 6). Steinberg (1996) developed a Structured Clinical Interview for the DSM-IV: Dissociative Disorders-Revised (SCID-D-R). Horevitz (1996) described the goal of treatment as the integration of cognitive function, affective experiences, a sense of personal history, and the personal environment, and not the fusion or integration of separate personalities. From a clinical standpoint, the integration of cognitive, emotive, and behavioral experiences is more practical.

The ISSD recommends an average of two treatment sessions per week over a three to five year time period for DID. An increase in the frequency of treatment and hospitalization is common when the DID client experiences setbacks.

The beginning of boundary management is important during this phase, and theorists and clinicians argue that DID clients are often victims of child abuse and neglect and they have grown up in situations where personal boundaries were not established or they were invaded. The clinician has to establish boundaries with the host and the alternate personalities. For example, DID clients are prone to crises, and the therapist has to make clear statements about his or her availability in emergencies, especially through telephone contacts. Specifically, unlimited telephone contact can lead to the DID client not recognizing that the therapist has a distinct life that has boundaries that are separate from the therapist's role as a helper. When clear telephone boundaries are established, often the DID client will not recognize that boundaries should exist, and this process can be used to generalize the principal of boundaries to other areas of the client's life.

The **fourth** phase of treatment is the forming of a contract with the alternate personalities to attend therapy and to agree not to harm themselves or the body they share.

The **fifth** phase of treatment involves a history gathering with every alternate personality. This will allow the therapist to understand the origins, functions, and relationships that each alternate personality has with every other.

Phase **six** involves helping the alternate personalities solve their problems. This may involve discussing painful events and establishing clear limits.

During phase **seven** the therapist has to have a conceptualization of how the alternate personalities function. This will provide information about the structure of the client's personality.

Phase **eight** involves facilitating the communication among the alternate personalities via hypnosis. This will begin the initial foundation for the association of cognitive, emotive, and behavioral dimensions.

During phase **nine** the therapist encourages unity or blending of alternate personalities, in contrast to the earlier power struggle among alters.

Phase **ten** involves teaching the client how to cope and learn adaptive ways of functioning interpersonally and in dealing with stress.

During phase **eleven** the client needs to form social networks for support. In addition, it is important for the client to understand the boundaries and distinctions of themselves and their support networks.

Working through and supporting is part of phase **twelve**. The client needs continued support and reinforcement for treatment gains. In addition, often, clients will have cognitive distortions in the areas of fear, anger, terror, panic anxiety, and so on. Moreover, many clients will resort to self-destructive frenzies when they experience intense feelings of shame or traumatic memories. Also, teaching the client how to handle depression is an important part of this phase.

The **final** phase of treatment is follow-up. It is not uncommon for clients to be evaluated by a complete battery of psychological tests during the conclusion of therapy. In addition, the therapist can use telephone calls as a means of following the client's progress once therapy is terminated.

Postfusion Treatment

For DID clients, it is not uncommon for them to relapse within 2 to 24 months after achieving the integration of **B**ehavioral, **A**ffective, **S**ensation, and **K**nowledge dimensions (called the Braun's BASK model, Braun 1988). If the BASK dimensions are integrated, mental processes are stable (Richardson 1998); neither fusion nor integration is absolute, because partial relapses are possible and the discovery of other alters is possible; therefore, integration should not be viewed as sacrosanct (Kluft 1990).

Hypnosis Applications for DID

Finally, the goals of hypnotic treatment are similar to that of other fusion procedures; that is, the integration or partial integration of the client's cognitive, affective, behavioral, and so on experiences to the maximum extent possible. The reader can see Chapter 5 for a fusion treatment transcript for DID.

Summary

Kluft (1982, 1984, 1991) researched 33 clients who were diagnosed as DID and who had an average of 13.9 personalities, ranging from 2 to 86. He found that it took 21.6 months from the initial diagnosis of DID to integration. He reassessed clients at a minimum of 27 months after integration, and he found that 31 (94%) had not relapsed into DID and 25 (75.8%) did not display dissociative features.

Dissociative disorders are disruptions in consciousness, memory, identity, and perceptions of one's environment. These disorders have similar features to acute stress disorder, posttraumatic stress disorder, and somatoform disorders.

Because these disorders involve alterations in the subjective sense of consciousness and perceptions, clinically, hypnosis appears to be a possible treatment; however, with DID, experimental studies are not available that assess the effects of hypnosis.

Finally, even though trauma, dissociation, and hypnosis have low intercorrelations, it is not known if this link is linear or is a cause-effect one. The intercorrelation among these variables is probably an indirect relationship. In conclusion, definitive quantitative longitudinal data are needed that show how hypnosis, dissociation, and trauma are related.

Dissociative Disorders in Children

In terms of the diagnosis of disorders in children, Putnam (1994) and Richardson (1998) described how children can suffer from the same symptoms as adults—such as repression, dissociation, amnesic experiences, conversion symptoms, mood disorders, and so on. Tyson (1992) argued that the majority of children experiencing DID have amnesia, behavioral fluctuations such as rapid regressions, changes in handwriting, changes in style of dress, and personality changes (Reagor, Kasten & Morelli 1992).

Children meeting the diagnostic criteria of DID tend to refer to themselves in the third person (Putnam 1991), and they tend to have developmental issues and to use imaginary playmates as attributions of their behavior. Often, the imaginary playmate is blamed for sexual acting out. Sanders (1992) found that adults who were diagnosed with DID tended to report one or more imaginary playmates when they were between the ages of 2 and 13. Sanders also noted that adults with DID tend to maintain contact with their imaginary playmates. Conversion reactions and sleep disturbances that include self-mutilation, fluctuating physical complaints, and sleepwalking are features of dissociative disorder in children.

Finally, Reagor et al. (1992) found that auditory hallucinations that are experienced internally are also part of the symptoms of a dissociative disorder. In summary, amnestic episodes of time lost, precocious sexual behaviors, developmental issues, conversion symptoms, sleep disturbances, mood disorders, and auditory hallucinations are clues to diagnosing dissociative disorders in children.

Assessment of Dissociative Disorders in Children

Developmental factors complicate the tasks of assessing dissociative disorders in children (Braun & Sachs 1985; Richardson 1998). For example, the normal development of dissociation, such as fantasy play and imaginary playmates, can complicate the assessment of maladaptive dissociation. Therefore, assessments should include a comprehensive clinical interview, information about the child's developmental milestones, family functioning, precipitating factors, and possible traumatic experiences the child may have had (Hornstein 1993; Putnam 1994; Richardson 1998).

For clinicians who are interested in learning how to clinically interview children with dissociative disorders, it is important to first learn how to interview children who are not suspected of having dissociative disorders. This will help a clinician learn how to phrase questions about abstract concepts in a more age-appropriate and concrete manner. The most difficult abstract constructs to assess with children who are suspected of having dissociative disorders are time loss and amnesic episodes (Hornstein 1993; Kluft 1984).

Adjunctive procedures to clinical interviews often include play activities as a means for a child to communicate his or her affect and associations. Projective techniques, dollhouses, puppets, play, storytelling materials, coloring books, and watercolor are often part of this clinical process. Curiously, play therapy and other informal induction procedures can elicit dissociation and hypnosis. A clinician can easily elicit hypnosis with children; however, understanding the developmental issues of children complicates the use of hypnosis.

There are liability issues and precautions a clinician should take when interviewing children. First, children, like adults, can reconstruct memory in ways that do not corroborate with empirical facts. For example, this writer has worked with children who were repeatedly told stories that were not based on empirical reality, and over time, it is not uncommon for these children to assimilate repetitive stories into their memories; hence, one precaution in working with children is that leading questions can affect the way children respond during interviewing.

Specifically, leading and/or closed-ended questions should be avoided when assessing children (Kluft 1984; Richardson 1998). This precaution is extremely important from a legal or liability point of view, because of the complex issues regarding recovered memories of sexual abuse. Finally, a clinician would want to avoid controversial techniques with children who are experiencing dissociation, and if he or she is not skilled in techniques for assessing dissociation and hypnotic procedures, this lack of competence can create potential liability issues (Knapp & Vande Creek 1996). In closing, Richardson (1998) provided the following when assessing children who may have been traumatized: (a) establish clear boundaries, (b) carefully form diagnoses and differential diagnoses, (c) employ reliable and valid clinical techniques, (d) assess and study family dynamics, (e) carefully document the entire process, and (f) consult with other professionals.

Screening Instruments for Dissociative Disorders with Children

There are two broad categories for instruments to screen dissociation with children, there are observer checklists such as the 17-item Child/Adolescent Dissociative Checklist (CADC; Reagor et al. 1992), and there are instruments completed by the child, such as the 28-item Children's Perceptual Alterations Scale (CPAS; Evers-Szostak & Sanders 1992).

One observer checklist, Child Dissociative Checklist (CDC), has been extensively evaluated. The **CDC** has good test-retest reliability, construct validity, and criterion-related validity (Putnam et al. 1993; Richardson 1998). Specifically, Putnam et al. reported a mean split-half reliability of .750 for the CDC and a median split-half reliability of .710. These reliability measures were obtained across several samples. Moreover, the mean and median Cronback's alphas were .835 and .800, respectively, for Putnam et al. data on the CDC. Finally, the test-retest coefficients of individual scale items for the CDC ranged from .57 to .92, and these data had a median test-retest coefficient of .735, $p = .0001$ (Richardson, 1998). Finally, the CDC is appropriate for children between 6 and 14 years of age (Putnam et al. 1993).

The CPAS is appropriate for children between the ages of 8 and 12 years of age (Evers- Szostak & Sanders 1992), and it has a mean and median split-half reliability across several studies of .745 and .750, respectively.

To summarize, there are several screening instruments that can be used to assess dissociation with children. Due to the difficulty in obtaining representative samples of children for many of these instruments, they can be best viewed as tools for assessments rather than formal psychological instruments. Finally, there is a need to replicate the results obtained with these screening tools with larger samples.

CHAPTER SUMMARY

Dissociative disorders are disruptions in consciousness, memory, and sense of identity that can affect adults and children. Conceptually, dissociative disorders overlap with acute stress disorder, PTSD, and somatoform disorders, so treatments that ameliorate these previously mentioned disorders should theoretically affect dissociative disorders. Clinically, hypnotic fusion techniques, regressive procedures, ego-strengthining techniques, anxiety and stress techniques, and psychoanalytic techniques are useful for dissociative and related disorders.

Chapter 5

TREATMENT

CHAPTER OVERVIEW

THIS CHAPTER STARTS by describing how to prepare clients for hypnosis, and it presents hypnotic screening instruments or tests that can be used to help determine if hypnosis is appropriate for a client. Moreover, the ingredients of a hypnosis transcript are also provided.

Next, a case presentation is used to show how a clinician can implement hypnosis. Moreover, the following hypnosis treatment transcripts are provided: direct hypnosis; indirect hypnosis; cognitive-behavioral hypnosis; psychodynamic hypnosis; postfusion treatment for DID; dissociative hypnosis; age progression hypnosis; regressive hypnosis; hypnosis for pain control; hypnosis for anxiety and stress; ego-strengthening hypnotic induction; unipolar depression hypnotic induction; and hypnosis for smoking cessation, weight loss, and rehabilitation. Finally, the chapter ends with a discussion of possible negative sequelae of hypnosis.

PREPARATION OF A CLIENT FOR HYPNOSIS

Clinicians should be aware that if they cannot treat a disorder without hypnosis, then hypnosis should not be employed, because hypnosis is only an adjunctive procedure and not a complete therapy in and of itself.

Clients should be educated about hypnosis. **First,** I usually point out that hypnosis is an adjunctive procedure, not a complete therapy in and of itself. **Second,** I state that there are different types of hypnosis, such as guided imagery, cognitive-behavioral, Ericksonian, and so forth. **Next,** I tell clients that all hypnosis is essentially self-hypnosis. **Furthermore,** I describe to clients how imagery and relaxation can lead to hypnosis. It is important to address clients' misconceptions about hypnosis, such as loss of consciousness, the weakening of the will, the giving away of secrets, and the inability to be dehypnotized. I stress with clients that nothing can occur through hypnosis that they do not want to happen.

Finally, I describe some everyday notions of hypnosis, such as driving and not being aware of how many miles one has driven, or becoming absorbed in a television show, movie, or book. Clinically, even though it has not been demonstrated experimentally, absorption is a feature of hypnosis. In closing, I describe some uses of hypnosis such as for the treatment of trauma, anxiety, personality disorders, unipolar depression, dissociative disorders, ego-strengthening, sexual disorders, nail-biting, obesity, smoking, and pain control.

Another way of preparing a client for hypnosis is through the use of Levels I and II psychotherapy skills (Sapp 1997b). **Level I psychotherapy skills** are designed to help a client to explore his or her emotions. This phase of psychotherapy involves paraphrasing statements back to the client.

For example, "You are feeling nervous about hypnosis. You are not sure of what will happen during hypnosis. You have some fear about hypnosis." It is important to reassure clients that uncertain or apprehensive feelings toward hypnosis are natural. And it is important to emphasize that anxiety, nervousness, apprehension, and so forth, are signs of intelligence and that you expect that hypnosis will be helpful. The hallmark of this phase of psychotherapy is to respond to clients' feelings, which can lead to clients experiencing genuineness and respect. The most important phase of Level I is responding to clients' feelings and the content that they communicate. Finally, this is also called the exploration phase of psychotherapy.

Level II, also called integrative understanding, is where clients continue to process information through the counseling process, and the counseling relationship gets stronger. The psychotherapist uses several psychotherapy skills during this phase such as summarizing content communicated by the client, challenging skills, and so on. The highlight of this stage is the psychotherapists' ability to help clients to establish goals for hypnosis. When a client has been prepared for hypnosis, hypnotic screening tests can be used to determine the client's ability to respond to hypnosis.

HYPNOTIC SCREENING TESTS

After a client has been prepared for hypnosis, and an effective psychotherapeutic relationship has been established, the client can be screened for hypnotic susceptibility. The two tests that will be described are the handclasp test and hand levitation tests. These screening tests are not the same as a standardized measure of hypnotizability, and the reader can consult Chapter 6 for a discussion of standardized hypnotizability measures. However, the reader may remember from other chapters that hypnotizability is not an all-or-none construct, but it exists on a continuum. For example, correlates of hypnotizability include, but are not limited to, ideomotor responding (motor responses that are the result of suggestions); cognitive capacities (imagery, dreams, age regression, and hyperamnesia); sensory denial or negation (analgesia, negative hallucinations); perceptual distortions of reality (positive hallucinations, hyperesthesia or increased sensitivity to touch, and alterations in meanings); and posthypnotic suggestions (amnesia and responses to hypnosis) (Sapp 1997a;1997d). The following is an induction script for the handclasp hypnotic screening test. Once you begin reading the script, descend your voice and read slowly and watch your client's nonverbal behavior.

Handclasp Hypnotic Screening Test

Whenever you are ready to elicit hypnosis, please get into a relaxed position. Close your eyes. When you are ready to initiate hypnosis, clasp your hands tightly together in front of your body. If you have your hands clasped together, begin to exert tension in that area. That's it, feel the force straining from both of your arms. In a little while, your hands, arms, and shoulders will tire from the strain and want to relax. It will feel difficult for your fingers and hands to come apart. It will feel as if they are stuck together.

Just to allow you to feel more relaxed and force your hands to feel tightly glued or stuck together, I will count down from ten to one. I will continue talking until it is time to terminate hypnosis. Now, ten . . . nine . . . eight . . . seven . . . six . . . five. A complete person in every way. Four . . . three . . . two . . . and one. Now, it is up to you, at your own rate of pace. Imagine that your hands are stuck together. And, yes, try, yes, try to pull them apart. Listen, just try . . . good. You can stop imagining that your hands are stuck together. Now, to show you that all hypnosis is self-hypnosis, I will say the word "now." When I say this word, you will begin to count to yourself from 1 to 10. As the numbers increase, you will feel yourself becoming more and more alert. When you say the number 10 to yourself, you will open your eyes and terminate hypnosis, feeling alert, refreshed, and comfortably relaxed. Whenever you go to sleep, you will really be able to enjoy the comfort of your bed. You are going to have a deep restful sleep, like the one you had a long . . . long . . . time ago. When you awaken, you will feel calm, secure, rested, comfortable, and confident. Yes, confident in your ability to easily go into and come out of hypnosis and to comfortably carry out your treatment. Easier and easier. "Now," it is up to you at your own pace and rate.

Debriefing

Discuss with your client the reactions that he or she had to hypnosis. If the client's hands remained clasped, he or she is probably responsive to hypnosis. Also, compare your observations with the client's inner subjective experiences. Another hypnotic screening test is the hand levitation test, and the following section presents the induction for this test.

Hand Levitation Hypnotic Screening Test

Get into a relaxed position if you would like to elicit hypnosis. Make a tight fist with either hand. I want you to make your fist as tight as possible. Focus all of your tension from the day onto your hand. Stare at the back of your hand. I just want you to pay close attention to your hand. As you pay attention to your hand, you can almost feel the blood flow through it. It may feel warm and tingly. That's it. Bring your attention to your hand.

Whenever you are ready to have a pleasant hypnotic experience, mobilize that tension in your body into your hand. I want you to feel that tension move from the tip of your head to the bottom of your feet. Let all the tension and energy focus in your shoulder, arm, and hand. That's right. Keep staring at your hand. While you are staring at it, notice what is happening; you experience yourself eliciting hypnosis. Let your hand tire from the struggle and loosen its grip. What was once steel is becoming like a soft stick of butter melting. I do not know how much tension is in your body, but there is plenty of time . . . plenty of time. Melting like butter. You are doing this at your own pace and rate.

In a few moments, I will count from one to ten. As I am counting your arm will raise. When I say the number ten, your arm will be floating in the air. Now, one . . . two . . . three . . . rising, floating . . . four . . . five. . . . Your arm is floating in the air. It is six. . . seven . . . rising . . . eight . . . nine, and ten. Now it is up to you, at your own rate and pace.

Now you can slowly let your arm descend and come out of your experience feeling refreshed and relaxed. It is almost as if you had just experienced a very peaceful nap. Whenever you go to sleep, you will have a very deep and restful sleep. It may be like the one you had a long time ago. Now you can terminate hypnosis feeling calm, secure, rested, comfortable, and confident. "Well," it is up to you at your own rate and pace.

Debriefing

Get your client to discuss his or her hypnotic experience. If your client's arm levitated, he or she is possibly responsive to hypnosis. Furthermore, compare your observations to your client's inner experiences. The case presentation that follows illustrates how to apply hypnosis.

CASE PRESENTATION

This case presentation concerns a 43-year-old married woman with a 15-year-old daughter. The client entered psychotherapy because of extreme anxiety. Let us refer to this client as Mary. Mary has been married to the same man for over 20 years. Throughout that period, she experienced severe unipolar depression. She has a low evaluation of herself, and she relies, almost entirely, on her husband to direct her life. For example, because Mary fears disapproval, she fears expressing her ideas or opinions to her husband.

Mary had the following DSM-IV multiaxal diagnosis:

Axis I   300.02   Generalized Anxiety Disorder
Axis II 301.6   Dependent Personality Disorder
Axis III   None
Axis IV   Problem with primary support group
Axis V GAF = 40

The goals of psychotherapy were to reduce the client's anxiety level and to work on ego-strengthening procedures. Mary requested hypnosis; therefore, I prepared her for hypnosis, and I gave her the handclasp hypnotic screening test. Mary responded well, and I gave her a form of hypnosis that was developed to help her reduce anxiety and to assist with ego-strengthening. The following is the transcript I used with Mary.

"Close your eyes and relax. Now I can talk to you in a special way, and you can process things at a deep level. I would like to communicate to your true self. There are some things I want you to remember. First, there is no need to feel annoyed either inwardly or outwardly. Second, stop suppressing your anger. Third, be aware of when you are impatient. Fourth, learn to overlook unimportant people, places, and things that used to annoy you, but do not be afraid to speak up patiently. If you start seeing a great deal of your resentment bubbling to the surface, do not be afraid. Remember not to analyze your feelings, but observe and release them. Actually, your resentment hurts you more than the cruel things that others do or say to you. You are going to learn how to overlook unimportant things and to be outspoken about things you need to be outspoken about.

"If you can be patient and see people the way they really are, you will be better off. Learn to be calm, patient, and not upset. You are going to learn that it is not possible to please people, and you will learn to stop trying. Criticism will roll off your back. It will be just like water rolling off the back of a duck. You will find yourself not being excited by praise or criticism.

"Every day your mind and body will become more relaxed, calm, placid . . . and more tranquil. You are going to find yourself becoming less easily worried . . . less fearful . . . and less apprehensive. Yes, every day you will become more and more physically fit. You are going to find yourself being more alert . . . more refreshed . . . more energetic . . . and more peaceful. Your nerves are going to become stronger and steadier. Yes, they will become steadier and stronger. Each and every day you are going to think more clearly. You will be able to concentrate more easily. You will be able to see events in their true perspective without blowing them out of proportion.

"Every day you can allow yourself to become emotionally

calmer ... more settled ... and not easily disturbed. You are going to find that life has a purpose, and you are going to have a sense of safety and security. These things will happen. You will feel happier, content, cheerful, optimistic, less easily discouraged, less easily depressed, and less anxious.

"Hypnosis will give you the courage to delete the **t** from **can't** and find that you can. If you expect positive things to happen, eventually, they will happen. Hypnosis will give you the ability to cope with the tension and stress of everyday living. You will be able to modify yourself to your environment, even if you cannot change your environment.

"As a way of terminating this experience, I will now count from one to five. Whenever you go to sleep, you will really be able to enjoy the comfort of your bed. You will have a very deep and restful sleep, and when you awaken you will feel calm, secure, and rested. Now, one ... two ... three ... four ... , and five. Now it is at your own rate and pace; it is up to you."

Case Presentation Summary

After four sessions with hypnosis, Mary reported decreases in her anxiety and depression. Furthermore, she stated that her ego-strength had increased—along with a greater reliance on herself. In closing, Mary indicated that changes had occurred within her marriage and that she had hope for the future. The ingredients of a hypnosis transcript is the focus of the next section.

INGREDIENTS OF HYPNOSIS TRANSCRIPTS

There are several ingredients of a hypnosis transcript. First, there is the **preinduction talk** that includes preparing the client for hypnosis and discussing the misconceptions of hypnosis. **Second,** many hypnosis inductions use some form of **progressive relaxation** such as breathing exercises, muscle-tension relaxation exercises, or guided imagery. The reader should note that alert hypnosis or hyperempiria can be elicited without relaxation instructions or suggestions. And there is some literature that suggests that alert hypnosis can be useful in treating attention deficit disorder and unipolar depression (Barabasz & Barabasz 1996). Commonly, another feature of hypnosis transcripts is **counting procedures** such as "you will find yourself entering hypnosis as I count from five to one." There are ego-strengthening exercises, such as "every day you will find yourself feeling stronger and stronger, more and more alert, and with less anxiety."

Finally, many transcripts contain **termination suggestions** such as "as I count from one to five you will come out of hypnosis feeling alert, refreshed, and you will not have any negative aftereffects." In terms of hypnosis transcripts, there are many styles such as direct hypnosis, indirect hypnosis, cognitive-behavioral hypnosis, psychodynamic hypnosis, dissociative hypnosis, regressive hypnosis, and so on.

DIRECT HYPNOSIS

Direct hypnosis uses direct and straightforward suggestions. This is the traditional view of hypnosis. Often, direct suggestions for progressive relaxation and guided imagery are part of the ingredients of direct hypnosis. Direct hypnosis is preferable for pain control. Hypnotic depth can be increased by counting or by offering direct suggestions for depth and heaviness.

Direct Hypnosis Transcript

Please close your eyes. I would like for you to concentrate on your breathing. Pay attention to your breathing. That's it. Notice as your diaphragm goes up and down, you become more and more relaxed. Can you remember a time when you were really relaxed? Remember what it was like to relax. Yes . . . allowing your mind and body to relax. Imagine being in a relaxed place.

Perhaps you will choose a place that is outside. Maybe you will choose a vacation spot. I do not know, but the place is completely up to you. Think about a very relaxing experience. Try to reexperience it now as though it is real again. I know some individuals who feel relaxed sitting by and looking into a fireplace, and others feel relaxed after or while exercising. I am not sure of the experience you will choose, but you are choosing one now.

Focus in on this experience. And just to help you relax more, I will count from five to one. Now, five . . . four . . . three . . . two . . . and one. I am going to show you how to use your arm as a lever to enter hypnosis. Make a tight fist with either hand and extend it straight out in front of your body. I want you to make your fist and arm as tight as possible. Focus all of the tension from the day into your hand. Pay attention to the heaviness that is developing in your hand. Notice that feeling. You can almost feel blood flow through your arm and hand. Whenever you are ready to elicit hypnosis, just simply allow your arm and hand to descend. That's it. Allowing your arm to slowly descend. As your arm goes down, you slowly enter hypnosis. That's fine ... entering hypnosis. I will again count from five to one, just to allow you to feel more relaxed and for your arm to feel very . . . very . . . heavy. Now, five . . . four . . . three . . . two . . . and one. Now, if your arm has not gone down by itself, let it go down.

I want to test your ability to respond to imagery. I want you to imagine that a balloon is attached to your arm. Yes, imagine that a balloon is causing your arm to slowly rise in the air. And to help you with this process, I will count from one to five. As the numbers increase, your arm will rise in the air more and more. Now, one . . . two . . . three . . . four . . . and five. Letting your arm rise in the air.

Now it is time to terminate hypnosis. I will count from six through ten as a means of ending this process. When I say the number ten, you will open your eyes and terminate this process feeling alert, refreshed, and comfortably relaxed. Whenever you go to sleep, you will really enjoy the comfort of your bed. You will have a deep, restful sleep, like ones you had a long . . . long . . .

time ago. When you awaken, you will feel calm secure, rested, comfortable, and confident. Yes, confident in your ability to use hypnosis. Now, six . . . seven . . . eight . . . nine, and ten. Easier and easier. It is up to you at your own rate and pace.

INDIRECT HYPNOSIS

Indirect hypnosis is based on indirect suggestions or suggestions worded in a permissive style. For example, permissive verbs such as "can" and "may" are used in contrast to more direct verbs such as "will" and "must." Some other names for indirect hypnosis are Ericksonian hypnosis and naturalistic hypnosis.

Indirect Hypnosis Transcript

Get as comfortable as you wish in that chair, or wherever you have yourself positioned. I am going to demonstrate a relaxation technique you can use to develop a very deep and pleasant hypnotic experience. Whenever you are ready to enter a relaxed state, clasp your hands together tightly in front of your body (the therapist should model this behavior).

Once you have them clasped together, begin to exert tension in that area. That's it. This time you will feel the force straining from both of your arms. In a little while your hands, arms, shoulders, and eyes will tire from the strain and want to relax. It will feel difficult for your fingers and hands to come apart. It will feel as if they are stuck together, but they will begin to come apart. That's it. As they do, you will correspondingly feel your eyes blinking and then eventually closing and then your hands will rest in your lap. This is very relaxing to say the least. This very pleasant feeling will travel throughout your body. It may appear that blood is streaming throughout your entire body. This can produce a warm, tingly, relaxing effect.

Of course, I will guide you throughout this process. At times, it may feel as if my voice corresponds to the pattern of your relaxation and matches the rhythm of your breathing; that's fine. Just to help you become more relaxed, I will count down from ten to one. I will continue talking until it's time for you to come out of this trance feeling very, very good....

Now, ten ... nine ... eight ... seven ... six ... five ... four ... three ... two and one. Now it is up to you at your own pace and rate. Good!

I want you to enjoy feeling comfortable.... Yes, that delightful feeling of relaxation spreading through the muscles of your face, neck, back, stomach, legs, and feet ... floating downward through your shoulders ... back ..., melting like butter.... If you want, you can allow yourself to melt like butter in that chair. (Adjust the wording to fit the position the client is in.) Allow the chair to hold you, feel the peacefulness, and comfort which is moving down through your stomach, thighs, legs, and toes. You are becoming more and more relaxed. If at any time you need to adjust your posture, feel free, because I would like you to enjoy feeling very comfortable. Yes ... have you noticed how deeply relaxed you are? (Adapted from Erickson 1976.) You probably have realized that the rhythm of your breathing has changed. It is slower, it is comfortable, and it is a good rhythm.

Now I would like to explain something to you. When you first went to school and learned to recognize numbers and letters, you didn't know it at that time that you were learning those numbers and letters for all the rest of your life. You formed a mental picture of those numbers and you formed mental visual pictures that would stay with you the rest of your life. You learned to form a mental visual picture of each letter of the alphabet without thinking about the fact that you would keep the visual image the rest of your life. In looking at that spot in your mind you have chosen, you have already formed a visual mental picture.

As I talk to you, you can keep right on looking mentally at that picture. As I talk to you, if you want, you can hear any sounds that you wish (mention any sounds in the environment). Actually, the only important thing for you is the sound of my voice and the meaning of what I have to say to you, so you do not really need to give attention to anything else unless you have a particular interest in the sounds in the room (mention any other things in the environment).

Now I will discuss your problem, and I will do it in this way. I will sketch it in general, and I want you to realize that I am only going to ask you to do things that you are capable of doing. There are many things we can do of which we are unaware. We can attend a lecture and because the lecturer is so interesting and stimulating, we do not even notice the passage of time. We are just interested in what the lecturer is saying.

If we attend a lecture that is dull, boring, and tiresome, one would feel the hardness of the seats. Yet, it could be the same seat in which one could sit and listen to an interesting lecturer and never feel all the discomforts and distress of not moving and the hardness of a seat. With a good lecturer, you don't even hear anything except his or her voice. Now you are here to listen to me. You are here to do certain things. In your lifetime of experience you have felt things and you have not felt some things that you could have felt if you had paid attention to them (confusional technique). You have had much experience in forgetting things that would seem, upon ordinary thinking, to be unforgettable.

For example, you were introduced to someone and you reply, "I am very pleased to meet you," but later you cannot (a change in tense in order to change the client's sense of time) remember the person's name. You have forgotten it just as fast as you heard it. In other words, you can do any of the things that I will ask of you. You know how to move. You also know how not to move. You can lower your blood pressure, yet you don't know how you do that. You can slow down your heartbeat, but you don't know how you do that; but all of the things I ask you do to, every one of them, will be within the range of your experiences, so just listen carefully, knowing that I will ask of you only those things that I know you can do.

First of all, I want you to enjoy feeling very comfortable. In fact, you can enjoy yourself so much that you can let your unconscious mind listen to me while your conscious mind can relax or busy itself with thoughts about things far removed from us, because many of the things that I want to assist you in accomplishing are governed by your unconscious mind. So now, continue as you are, at ease, in comfort, and at the proper time, I will give you all the directions necessary for you to take care of your problems, all of those you need to deal with.

If one were to ask the question, "What would you ask for if you were granted one wish?" I'm sure your answer would vary. (Adapted from Masters 1978.) Some people would ask for a house, others would ask for a car. Others may ask for health, while yet others may ask for education. Maybe you would ask for money . . . or maybe you would ask for a long life, but in reality, ambition can be one's opportunity in life. If one were truly in tune with reality, I'm sure one would choose quite differently. For example, why not wish that everything that you have ever wished will become true? Here you would be using one wish to build the foundation for other wishes. Everyone has this choice in life, but one cannot make it when things are hidden from view.

I once heard a story about a king named Solomon. He was granted one single wish. King Solomon wished for an understanding heart. Since he had a propensity toward humanity, his wish was granted. King Solomon was given fame, honor, riches, and everything one's heart could desire. (Adapted from Bassman 1983.) That's it, allow yourself to relax more and more . . . . In a little while, I am going to ask you to imagine a bright, intense beam of light shining directly into your eyes. Perhaps you will tell yourself it is glaring sunlight shining into your eyes. Whatever you imagine or tell yourself, you will remember what it feels like as glaring, bright lights shine directly in your eyes. It is, of course, very difficult to open your eyes as you imagine this.

Well, I am going to ask you to try to open your eyes as you imagine this. Yes, to try to open your eyes, but you will not be able to do so. Yes, the harder you try to open your eyes the more they will stay closed.

So imagine and tell yourself that a bright ray of glaring, bright light is shining directly in your eyes, glaring, bright light directly in your eyes. . . . Now, try, yes, try to open them, but you will not be able to because the harder you try, the more they will want to stay closed. Try, try in the glaring light. (After about ten seconds, say the following.) All right, you can relax. You did fine. Now, as you relax deeply, you can allow the relaxation from the light to warmly relax your entire body. Let the light disappear. It went behind the clouds. Relax . . . you have demonstrated by the ability of your mind that you can exert control over your body. Good! You have within yourself the ability to relax . . . to imagine . . . and to utilize your own inner resources to control your physiological processes.

As you remain deeply in a trance, open your eyes. Open your eyes now! The intense light is gone. That's fine. Just look around the room and pick some spot to look at steadily as you continue to relax deeply with your eyes open. Look at any spot there . . . and do not touch it. Yes, just keep looking at that spot. Now there is no need to talk. No need to move. You really don't need to pay attention to me because your unconscious mind will hear me, and it will understand. You really don't need to pay attention to me.

While you have been sitting there, you've been doing the same thing that you did when you first went to school. Remember when you first learned the task of writing the letters of the alphabet. It seemed like an impossible task ... and how do you recognize a "b?" How is it different from a "d"? Numbers: is a 6 an upside down 9, or is a 9 an upside down 6 . . . while you were mastering those problems, you were forming mental images that would stay with you for the rest of your life. No, you did not know it then, but while you were sitting there the same thing has been happening to you now happened to you then.

Your respiration has changed. Your blood pressure has changed, and you have a mental image, a visualized image of that spot and now you may project on that spot, your favorite relaxing place, as you close your eyes, now!

Now you can enjoy the comfort of going even deeper into the trance. I want you to enjoy every moment of it . . . , and you can have a lot of pleasure in becoming aware of the comforts . . . within yourself. One of those is the understanding you can go back, and perhaps you might have the experience of sensing as you rest and relax . . . the incredible healing forces at work . . . restoring . . . nourishing . . . improving your memory . . . improving your health. If distracting thoughts enter your mind, do not fight them. Be aware of these thoughts.

Now listen to me! There is a way to cope and change this scenario into a pleasant one. You can relax deeply at your own pace. (Adapted from Masters 1978.) Let thoughts rise! Don't try to suppress them. Most people are accustomed to thinking with their feelings and becoming lost in them. Many people are used to living in a daydream state of escape. You have the power to escape this daydream or negative state. You may be saying to yourself, now, when I see him or her I will say this or that. Stop planning discussions! Let everything be spontaneous. Each time you do this exercise you will be creating an increased ability to observe and thereby control your thoughts from within yourself. This will be—not because I say so, but because this exercise will make it so.

Each time you do this exercise it will create a greater awareness of the present and the unpleasant events of the past will become less important and dissolved in the light of reality. If you like, focus your attention on your breathing and recognize how easily deep breathing alone can help to produce a nice state of gentle relaxation. Let your body breathe by itself, according to its own natural rhythm. Slowly . . . easily . . . and deeply. . . . Whatever you feel, is your body's way of acknowledging the experience of relaxation, comfort, and peace of mind.

Remember your breathing . . . , slowly and deeply. As you concentrate your attention on your breathing, give your body a few moments to relax deeply and fully. Feel all the tension, tightness, or discomfort draining away, down your spine, down your legs, and into the ground. With each breath, you may be surprised to feel yourself becoming more and more deeply relaxed . . . comfortable . . . and at ease. Enjoy this nice state of relaxation.

(Adapted from Hartland 1971.) Every day . . . you will become physically stronger and fitter. You will become more alert . . . more wide awake . . . more energetic. You will become much less easily tired . . . and less easily fatigued . . . much less easily tired . . . much less easily fatigued . . . much less easily discouraged. Every day, your nerves will become stronger and steadier. You will become so deeply interested in whatever is going on . . . that your mind will become much less preoccupied with yourself.

Every day, you will become emotionally much calmer . . . much more settled . . . much less easily disturbed. Every day, you will feel a greater sense of awareness for the present and events of the past will become less and less meaningful. Every day . . . you will feel a greater feeling of personal safety and security . . . than you have felt for a long, long time. Every day . . . you will become . . . and you will remain . . . more and more completely relaxed . . . both mentally and physically.

All of these things will happen . . . exactly as I say they will happen . . . you are going to feel much happier . . . much more contented . . . much more cheerful . . . much more optimistic . . . much less easily discouraged . . . much less easily depressed. As you relax and enjoy how wonderful it feels to be comfortable, peaceful, and at ease . . . tell yourself that you can return any time you wish . . . simply by letting go and taking a few moments to relax yourself and letting your imagination carry you there. . . . Each time you come to visit, you will find it even more beautiful, more serene, and more peaceful as new horizons are opened for you to experience. It is so easy . . . so accessible . . . so available to you, even when you are no longer with me, my voice will be with you . . . it will be the voice of a member of your family . . . it will be the voice of the wind . . . the rain . . . and, yes, the voice of the sun . . . . You will remember that the secret lies within you.

Just to show you that you can achieve what you set out to, and that you are able to use hypnosis to help yourself, in a few moments, I will say the word "now." When I say this word, you will begin to count to yourself from one to ten. As the numbers increase, you will feel yourself becoming more and more alert. When you say the number ten to yourself, you will open your eyes and come out of the trance feeling alert, refreshed and also very comfortably relaxed . . . and whenever you go to sleep, you will really be able to enjoy the comfort of your bed. You will have a very deep and restful sleep, like one you had a long . . . long . . . time ago. When you awaken, you will feel calm and secure, rested, comfortable, and confident. Yes, confident in your ability to easily go into and come out of a trance, and to comfortably carry out this treatment, easier and easier. "Now," it is up to you, at your own pace and rate. Good.

Debriefing

It is important to get your client to summarize his or her experiences. This helps the client to process the experience, and it allows the client to continue to dehypnotize.

COGNITIVE-BEHAVIORAL HYPNOSIS (CBH)

Cognitive-behavioral hypnosis (CBH) is a term for combining hypnosis with cognitive- behavioral strategies. One assumption of this approach is that psychological problems are the result of negative self-hypnosis (Araoz 1981, 1982, 1985). This is similar to the principles emphasized by Ellis (1993), who stated that emotional disturbances are the result of irrational thinking. The CBH approach is a nonstate theoretical approach. The transcript that follows is a CBH one.

CBH Transcript

Get into a relaxed position, close your eyes, and I will show you how to elicit cognitive-behavioral hypnosis within yourself. First, I would just like you to relax. You can relax by just thinking about relaxation. Use your thoughts to relax your mind, which in turn will relax your body. Learning to use cognitive-behavioral hypnosis involves controlling your thinking and attention. Thinking is the things we say to ourselves. Thinking or using your mind is the first step toward change.

We can talk more about thinking. Many of our thoughts are

based on the ways we think about social situations. Often, social situations such as public speaking and so on do not produce anxiety, but it is the way we look or think about social situations that produce anxiety and fear. For example, some students who have difficulty in school will tell themselves that negative things are going to happen, that they are not good, and the result is negative emotions. If you can get rid of self-defeating thoughts, all the musts, and other derivatives, you will be better off. You will be even better off if you can replace self-defeating thoughts with realistic ones.

Now let's proceed with cognitive-behavioral hypnosis. If the phone rings or if someone comes to the door, I will take care of it. The important thing for you is just relaxing. If you think about relaxation, your body will feel relaxed. And to help you, I will count from ten to one. As the numbers are going down, your level of relaxation will increase. Now, 10 . . . 9 . . . 8 . . . a full person in every way. It is 7 . . . 6 . . . 5 . . . 4 . . . 3 . . . 2 . . . 1.

Cognitive-behavioral hypnosis involves cognitively imagining a scene. In your mind's eye, imagine a very relaxing scene. You can choose a scene that is indoors or outdoors. Take your time and visualize every aspect of that scene. See it as clearly as possible. Notice the time of day or night. Yes, cognitive-behavioral hypnosis uses your imagination to produce changes in your inner experiences. Really let your imagination get into this scene . . . .

When I say the word "now," you will count to yourself from one to ten. When you say the number ten, you will come out of cognitive-behavioral hypnosis feeling relaxed, refreshed, and confident in your ability to use cognitive-behavioral hypnosis.

Debriefing

Have the client describe his or her experience and make adjustments in the transcript based on the client's comments.

PSYCHOANALYSIS AND HYPNOSIS

Erika Fromm

Both Erika Fromm and Michael Nash have similar, yet different ego **psychological theories of hypnosis** (Fromm & Nash 1997). Fromm acknowledges that her work is an adaptation of the theses of Gill and Brenman of the 1950s. Moreover, her work was influenced by Kris and Harmann of the 1930s, who elaborated on adaptive regression or regression in the service of the ego. That is, one is able to relax and go backward on the developmental ladder.

Actually, for Fromm, regression in the service of the ego is non-pathological, healthy, and short-term regression. Very similar to Edmonston (1981, 1991), Fromm sees hypnotic relaxation as an ego-modulated relaxation of defensive barriers that leads to a shift from secondary process thinking to primary process thinking. Fromm and Nash view hypnosis as a shift in cognitive processes and as an altered state of consciousness. In fact, creativity is a specific example of regression in the service of the ego.

There are four phases of creativity: (1) preparation, (2) incubation, (3) illumination, and (4) verification or evaluation. Incubation is the relaxation phase, and illumination is analogous to the regression in service of the ego, where unconscious material surfaces to consciousness.

Unlike some hypnosis theorists, Fromm believes that ego activity is linked with free will, defense, and mastery. And ego passivity is tied to feelings of being overwhelmed and the inability to cope. Interestingly, one critical point with Fromm's theory is that she defines ego activity in regard to the hypnotic state as a volitional mental activity.

Fromm defined **ego receptivity** as a generalized reality orientation in which consciousness has faded into the background of preconsciousness. During ego receptivity, how does the client feel? He or she feels a greater openness to experience stimuli, both internally and externally. And an intensified transference relationship develops during this process. In addition, active, goal-directed behavior, secondary processing (logical or ratiocinative) and voluntarism occur during the ego receptivity hypnotic phase, and finally the client "just lets go." Now, the client is more open to hypnotic suggestions and preconscious and unconscious material surface to awareness. In closing, for ego receptivity to occur, the client must have trust in the therapist.

Attention, absorption, and the **general reality orientation (GRO)** are features of Fromm's theory. Obviously, attention and absorption are concepts that originate from cognitive psychology, and the GRO has been acknowledged as an important feature of hypnosis.

In regard to attention, Fromm describes concentrated or focused and expansive or free-floating forms of attention. With expansive attention, the client "lets go," and a variety of feelings, thoughts, memories, and so on enter into attentional awareness.

With her research on self-hypnosis, Fromm found that concentrated attention always correlates with ego activity, and expansive attention is associated with letting go and surrendering oneself to ego receptivity.

In contrast to cognitive psychologists, Fromm views attention and absorption as ego functions, and in her laboratory she has found two categories or variables that differentiate hypnosis from the waking state, structural and content. Structural factors characterize the nature of the hypnotic state and they include absorption, letting the GRO fade into the background of awareness, increased ego receptivity, expansive attention, and the subjective experience of a deep trance. Content categories or variables include increased imagery production, hyperamnesia, stronger affect, more enjoyable and more conflicting thoughts, hypnotic dreams, working on personal issues, and self-suggested ideomotor and ideosensory responding.

Michael Nash

Unlike Fromm, who views regression as temporal and topographic, Nash believes that regression in hypnosis is solely **topographic**. Even though Nash accepts regression as "in the service of the ego," he still views regression as topographic in nature. In support of Nash's view, hypnosis researches have failed to find any credible evidence that hypnosis brings back authentic childlike cognitive, psychological, perceptual, or physiological functionings. Similarly to Freud, Nash believes that hypnosis alters the equilibrium between primary and secondary process mentation in that there is more primary process, greater availability of affect, prevalence of condensation-displacement, body distortion, and changes in volitional experiences. One can infer from Nash's theory that hypnosis is related to fantasy, reverie, and dreaming.

To reiterate, Fromm views hypnosis as an inseparable temporal and topographic phenomenon. In contrast, Nash believes that associating hypnosis to earlier stages of psychological development is misleading, and the topographic nature of hypnosis is one of its forensic limitations. The following is a psychodynamic transcript.

PSYCHODYNAMIC HYPNOSIS TRANSCRIPT

Close your eyes and get into a relaxed position. We want to focus on bringing unconscious thoughts to conscious awareness. Yes, let your body and mind relax and try not to control your thoughts. Let your thoughts rise to the surface of your mind, while your body relaxes and lets go. This experience may remind you of an early childhood experience . . . or it may remind you of a person that you forgot. Maybe it reminds you of something forgotten . . . a sensation or an experience. Whatever it brings to your mind, do not resist it.

Yes, let thoughts rise and surface into conscious awareness. And to help you relax more, I will count from 5 to 1. As the numbers go down, your unconscious thoughts will increase their access to conscious awareness. Simultaneously, your body and mind will relax. Now, 5 . . . 4 . . . 3 . . . 2 . . . and 1. Let your unconscious thoughts continue to surface into conscious awareness. Do not censure any thoughts; just observe these thoughts objectively.

As thoughts surface to conscious awareness, it is like observing words on a screen. See them as clearly as you can. Do not try to touch or manipulate these words. Keep observing them. Yes, observe them one by one. Each word stimulating a thought . . . feeling . . . experience . . . sensation that you may have not thought about in a long time. Continue as you are, at ease . . . objective, and focusing on all of these experiences. Let as many thoughts surface as possible. . . .

By counting from 1 to 5, now, it is time to terminate this experience. But, first, I would like for you to focus on relaxing again, and this time letting your mind carry you to a very relaxing and peaceful place. Let your mind carry you to this place now. . . . Experience it as clearly as possible. Notice the time of day or night. This is a wonderful place. Yes, it is alive, and it gives you energy, the ability to focus, the ability to concentrate, and it gives you the ability to heal your mind and body.

You are going to notice differences in your mind and body. They will get stronger and stronger. Your mind will become more alert. Your concentration and memory will improve. These things will happen not because I say so, but your mind will make things come true.

As we terminate this process by counting from 1 to 5, just continue as you are. When the numbers increase, you will come out of this hypnotic trance feeling alert, refreshed, and energized. And whenever you go to sleep, you will really enjoy your sleep. Now, 1 . . . 2 . . . 3 . . . 4 . . . and 5. It is up to you. You are dehypnotizing at your own rate and pace.

Debriefing

It is important to process the unconscious images, thoughts, and feelings that your client reports. And it is important to help the client gain insight into how unconscious processes affect conscious awareness. The transcript that follows illustrates a hypnotic fusion technique for DID.

HYPNOTIC FUSION TECHNIQUE FOR DID

You may keep your eyes opened or you may close them. The purpose of this induction is to associate or fuse various aspects of your mind and body. Allow your mind to carry you to a very safe and relaxed place. Yes, a place where you feel secure and can communicate with various aspects of yourself. Of course, the person I am talking to and the other aspects of yourself have to give me permission to proceed. Let's allow a few moments for all aspects of yourself to understand what I am communicating. If there are any aspects of yourself that disagree with this fusion process, let that aspect speak now. . . .

Well, let's continue. Imagine viewing every aspect of yourself through an imaginary television screen. Notice every aspect of yourself moving closer and closer together. Of course, all of this is only occurring because each aspect of yourself wants this fusion process to continue. Notice how each and every feeling, memory, behavior, and so on are coming together. This process is the opposite of your dissociative process, for it is associative.

Be aware of every aspect of your mind moving closer and closer together. Just keep allowing your mind and body to become unified.

If you want, you can imagine that every aspect of yourself is in a very safe, relaxed, and special place. Every aspect of yourself is moving together toward an imaginary circle of unity. The closer they get within that circle, the more connected and whole you feel. It may appear that every aspect of yourself is communicating as one. Sense, feel, and be aware of this difference, and this process will continue after hypnosis has ended.

It is time to end hypnosis, but you will feel that the conscious and unconscious aspects of yourself are unifying. This process will continue for some time until you feel a greater sense of your unified self, and you will experience a greater sense of a very stable self.

Let us end this session of hypnosis by counting from 5 to 1. As the numbers decrease, you will come out of hypnosis feeling more whole and unified. Whenever you go to sleep, this association process will continue. That is, you will feel stronger each and every day. Your nerves will become stronger and your mind will become emotionally calmer. Finally, you will feel the integrative benefits of hypnosis every day. Now, 5. . . 4. . . 3. . . 2. . . and 1. It is up to you at your own rate and pace.

Debriefing

Because DID clients are particularly influenced by suggestions, it is important for the therapist to offer tentative hypotheses about aspects of the treatment that are unclear. Moreover, it is not uncommon for DID clients to have memories that emerge as a result of hypnosis; however, therapists should be careful and not accept clients' symbolic reality as actual reality, because DID clients' imaginations can produce memories. At this juncture of therapy, it is important to stay objective and to carefully employ levels I and II counseling skills. Finally, it is important to emphasize that fusion will continue and that it may be necessary for postfusion treatment strategies. In closing, the transcript that follows is a dissociation one.

DISSOCIATION TRANSCRIPT

Close your eyes. The purpose of this induction is to teach you how to mentally disconnect your mind from your body. First, allow your entire body to relax. If there is tension in your body, notice it and let it go. Relax your mind and body now. Yes, relax your head, shoulders, neck, back, legs, and feet. Allow your entire body to relax. Now let the tension go. That's it, feeling very relaxed. Imagine looking at yourself through a television screen. Observe yourself and notice how detached and removed you feel. It is like looking at another person, but the person you are observing is yourself. Now, notice how your body feels. It feels detached, disconnected, and dissociated. Continue this experience. Yes, observing yourself through an imaginary screen. Let yourself experience this process. It may feel like your conscious mind is disconnecting from your unconscious mind. One part of your mind can hear these words, but another part of your mind is processing things on a hidden level. Just let things happen. Try not to make things happen. Continue as you are, nicely dissociated and relaxed.

It is time to end this experience by counting from 1 to 5. As the numbers increase, you will slowly return to your natural state of mind. Yes, unified and reconnected. You will feel refreshed and energized. Now, 1 . . . 2 . . . 3 . . . 4 . . . and 5.

Debriefing

Process this experience with your client. Try to determine if the client experienced the process as involuntary. The following transcript demonstrates age progression.

AGE PROGRESSION TRANSCRIPT

This transcript is designed to get you to explore some of the possibilities of your future. So, close your eyes and get into a relaxed position. As your entire body relaxes, just let yourself let go of any tension and tightness that may be in your body. Of course, there is plenty of time . . . plenty of time. . . . There is no need to worry or think about anything else. Because you are in control, you can do some interesting things by projecting your mind into the future.

Easily, if you want, you can erase today's day and date out of your mind, and project yourself into the future. By counting forward, you can allow your mind to move into the future. Yes, exploring some future meanings and possibilities of your life. Now, mentally project yourself into the future. One . . . moving forward into your future. Two . . . forward . . . continuing into your future. Notice how your body ... environment . . ., and emotions are changing. Three . . . mentally, moving forward in time. Four

... continuing ... moving straight ahead in time. Altering time within your mind. Five ... continue to move forward ... forward ... forward in time. Six ... continue to move. Now, 7 ... 8 ... 9 ... and 10.

You have moved forward in time within your mind. Notice your feelings, your body, and your environment. As I watch you, the expressions on your face remind me of the passage of time. That is right, time has moved forward. Within your mind's eye, see how your life has changed. I wonder what is the status of your personal life? And I wonder where are you in terms of your career? I wonder where are you right now? Who are you with? You appear more mature ... secure, and comfortable with your life. As you continue this process, tell yourself that you do not have to be as affected by your past as you were some time earlier. Enjoy feeling free and refreshed for a few moments .... After a few moments, we will end this exercise. But, for now, enjoy your feelings and sensations.

It is now time to end this process by counting from 10 to 1. As I say the numbers, you will find yourself returning to the present. After I stop counting, you will continue moving backward in time until you are back to your current age. When I stop counting, you will remember the correct day and date. Now, 10 ... 9 ... 8 ... 7 ... 6 ... 5 ... 4 ... 3 ... 2 ..., and 1. You are back to your normal self.

Debriefing

Make sure that your client has dehypnotized and process with the client his or her experiences to the age progression. The next transcript demonstrates age regression.

AGE REGRESSION TRANSCRIPT

The purpose of this transcript is to return to an earlier period in your mind. Get into a relaxed position. Close your eyes and just relax. Relax your entire body by letting yourself feel heavy and limp. Yes, letting yourself feel comfortable and relaxed. Yes, you can feel heavy and limp. Feel more and more comfortable. Feel more and more relaxed. Just allow yourself to relax . . . relax . . . relax.

If you want, you can forget today's day and date. Think along these lines, and allow yourself to return to an earlier time that is pleasant and peaceful. We can count backward and allow you to return to an earlier time that is safe . . . peaceful . . . and pleasant. Yes, returning to a very safe place. This is a secure place. Now, 10 . . . going backward in time. Nine . . . returning to an earlier period of your life. Of course, this place is safe and comfortable. Eight . . . backward, backward in time. Notice the changes in your body . . . emotions . . . and the environment around you. Now, 7 . . . 6 . . . 5 . . . 4 . . . 3 . . . 2 . . . and 1.

You are now at an earlier period of your life. Pay attention to your emotions, your body, and the environment around you. As I watch you, it reminds me of one day when I was sitting in school. Often I would daydream when I became tired of listening to my teacher, or learning to decipher a p from a b. Numbers, I had trouble determining if a 6 was an upside down 9. But I was able to return to an earlier period within my mind. I could create whatever I wanted to create within my imagination. I could bring the warmest and most pleasant feelings. Take a few moments to enjoy this process. . . .

Now it is time to start terminating this process by counting from 1 to 10. As I say the numbers, you will find yourself increasing in size, and you will experience time moving forward. Once I stop counting, you will continue moving forward in time until you are back to your current age. When I stop counting, you will remember and know the correct day and date. Now, 1 . . . 2 . . . 3 . . . 4 . . . 5 . . . 6 . . . 7 . . . 8 . . . 9 . . . and 10. You are back to your normal way of functioning.

Debriefing

Make sure that your client has terminated hypnosis and process the experience with him or her. It should be noted that regressive hypnosis should only be used when it is clinically indicated. The next transcript deals with pain control.

IMPLICATIONS OF HYPNOSIS FOR PAIN CONTROL

Before using hypnosis to control pain, a clinician should have specialized training in the physiology of pain, and he or she should have supervised experience in pain management. Using hypnosis to control pain can be a complex process.

Hilgard's (1991, 1994) neodissociation theory appears to be the best explanation of how hypnosis controls pain; however, as Barber (1999) suggests (see Chapter 6), most of the clients Hilgard worked with were amnesic-prone; that is, they had an amnesia for pain, because they were aware of pain on an unconscious level (hidden observer), but they were not aware of pain on a conscious level. If Barber is correct, and I believe he is, researchers and clinicians see clients with different personality types.

For example, clients with a fantasy-prone personality are able to reinterpret pain through their fantasy ability. To illustrate, this personality style is able to think along with the clinician's suggestions; they are able to feel what is being suggested, and they are able to manipulate the meaning of pain through their fantasies.

Finally, clients who have positive-set or attitudes toward hypnosis are able to imagine changes in their pain, but unlike the amnesic-prone and fantasy-prone, these clients do not have the natural abilities of the previously mentioned types. Hence, using hypnosis to help clients control pain requires an assessment of a client's personality type, and the clinician must be aware of his or her personal dimensions such as empathy, directness, expertness, and so on. Finally, the last dimension that can affect pain are the kinds of suggestions given such as direct or indirect, and the tone of the clinician's voice can affect the way the client responds.

Pain Control Transcript

Close your eyes and relax. The purpose of this transcript is to show you how to manage your pain. Let's talk about your pain. Well, pain can be constant or sporadic, or it can be chronic or acute. I am not sure of the meaning of your pain, but it is possible to control it. I would like for you to imagine a bucket filled with an imaginary fluid. This fluid is a powerful analgesic in that it can remove or decrease pain. See that imaginary bucket in your mind's eyes. Let it be your favorite color. Imagine that it is filled with an imaginary fluid that can remove and decrease pain. Slowly raise your left or right hand and slowly dip it into the imaginary bucket. Slowly swirl or twirl your hand around in the bucket so that it can absorb as much of this fluid as possible. Let the fluid become absorbed deeply within your hand. Perhaps your hand is becoming warm and tingly. Allow this to happen for as long as you need. Once you are finished, put your hand on the part of your body that needs pain relief. You may be surprised at the amount of relief you feel as the magical fluid is transferred from your hand to that part of your body that is in discomfort.

Allow as much of the magical fluid to be transferred to the affected part of your body as possible. Now feel the difference in what was the painful part of your body. Perhaps that part of your body feels warm and numb . . . yes, warm and numb. . . . Let that part of your body become as numb as you want. Remember one thing about pain. It is a signal to your body, so I want a certain part of your mind, your unconscious, to process the meaning of your pain while your conscious mind will not have any memory of pain. Continue this process for as long as you need in order to obtain relief. When you are ready to end this process, just shake your hand and all sensations will return, but your relief from pain will continue. And each time you do this exercise you will get greater relief than the time before. Actually, each time you perform this exercise, you will get a greater sense of control of your pain. You will find that your pain has a different meaning. Whenever you are ready to end this process, just let yourself return to your natural state of mind. It is up to you at your own rate and pace.

Debriefing

Discuss with your client his or her reactions. Try to increase the client's expectations that his or her reactions can lead to pain control, and try to increase the client's expectations that his or her pain can be controlled. The focus of the next transcript is anxiety and stress.

ANXIETY AND STRESS

Anxiety or **stress** are affective disorders in which clients experience debilitating anxiety and/or stress. Research suggests that worry is the hallmark of anxiety disorders, and **worry** is viewed as a cognitive concern (Sapp 1997). In contrast, **emotionality**, which is another component of anxiety, is the physiological response that the body has to worry. Curiously, clients' worry cognitions tend to be automatic and habitual. The diagnosis of an anxiety disorder is made if anxiety affects a client's quality of life. Readers can consult the **Diagnostic and Statistical Manual of Mental Disorders** (1994, 4th ed.) for a thorough discussion of anxiety disorders. And Sapp (1999) provides a complete discussion of how to assess and treat anxiety disorders, especially test anxiety. Finally, since worry cognitions are automatic, clearly, the automaticity feature of hypnosis makes it a treatment of choice (see Chapter 6 for a discussion of hypnosis and automaticity).

Anxiety and Stress Transcript

This hypnotic induction will help you learn how to handle anxiety and stress. Close your eyes and get into a relaxed position. Think about a relaxed scene. As you are thinking about this scene, rate your anxiety and stress on a 1-to-10-point scale, where 1 is the lowest amount of anxiety, and stress and 10 is the maximum amount of anxiety. Wherever your current level of anxiety, let it decrease. Let your anxiety and stress level decrease now. Notice the difference between how you are able to relax, and how you were when you were tense. Yes, notice the difference between tension and relaxation.

I can help you to relax more by counting from 5 to 1. Now, 5 . . . becoming more deeply relaxed. Four, let go and just relax. Three, stop struggling and relax. Now it is two . . . and one. Be aware of your mental and physical relaxation.

There are some things you will notice each and every day. First, you will not be annoyed inwardly or outwardly. Second, you will notice differences in your levels of stress and anxiety. They will become less frequent and less severe. Yes, they will be less frequent and less severe until you have control of them. You will be able to manage your anxiety and stress.

Third, you will not experience the same level of stress and anxiety that you experienced yesterday. Fourth, actually, you will find that anxiety and stress are signals that you need to relax and let go.

Fifth, you will feel the benefits of hypnosis each day. You are going to feel more calm and secure. Yes, you will be more confident in your ability to use hypnosis to control your anxiety and stress.

Now you can end this process at your own rate and pace. Slowly dehypnotize yourself. You feel fine, alert, relaxed, and ready to use hypnosis to solve your problems.

Debriefing

Process the degree of relaxation the client experienced. Some clients will feel that tape recording this induction helps with the process of learning hypnosis. Ego-strengthening is the focus of the next induction.

Ego-Strengthening Induction Transcript

Please relax yourself any way you can. If you like, you can close our eyes and just relax by concentrating on your breathing. Some people relax by thinking about a relaxing scene. Others relax by just simply letting go. Let yourself relax. Yes, relax your head, face, neck, trunk, legs, and feet. Relax your entire body.

Now the purpose of this form of hypnosis is to strengthen your ego. Self-esteem involves the feelings you have about yourself, whereas self-concept is the mental picture of yourself. So see yourself, within your mind's eye, becoming physically stronger and stronger. See yourself becoming more and more energetic. Your nerves are getting stronger and steadier. Your mind will become stronger, calmer, composed, placid, and tranquil. Yes, each day your mind will become much calmer, clearer . . . composed . . . placid . . . and tranquil. You will become less easily worried . . . less easily agitated . . . much less fearful, and less easily upset. Every day you are going to find that you can stand on your own feet. You will find that you have more strength and confidence in yourself, not because I say so, but because this exercise of using your mind will make it so. Each day you will have a strong sense of confidence in yourself, your goals, and plans. Every day you will feel the benefits of hypnosis. Whenever you are ready to bring hypnosis to an end, just count to yourself from one to five. As the numbers increase, you will dehypnotize yourself and feel alert and refreshed. Now it is up to you.

Debriefing

Explore the process your client experienced and make adjustments based upon your client's experience. Unipolar depression is the focus of the next transcript.

UNIPOLAR DEPRESSION

Beck and Weishaar (1995) found that **cognitive therapy** was effective in treating unipolar depression—depression without a manic phase. Moreover, cognitive therapy was found to be superior or equal to antidepressant medication (Blackburn, Bishop, Glen, Whalley & Christie 1981; Dobson 1989).

Barabasz and Barabasz (1996) and Yapko (1996) reported that hypnosis is effective in treating unipolar depression. Theoretically, active-alert hypnosis (Barabasz & Barabasz 1996) and hyperemperia (Gibbons 1979), should be effective for unipolar depression. Essentially, hypnosis, like cognitive therapy, can be used to change clients' dysfunctional cognitions, especially automatic ones. The following transcripts illustrate this process.

Unipolar Depression Hypnosis Transcript

Please close your eyes. I want you to produce an active-alert process within yourself by becoming very ... very absorbed with my voice. As my voice increases in intensity, you will feel more mentally alert. Keep focusing on the quality of my voice. (The therapist should speak in a loud and focused tone.)

To increase your mental activity, I will now quickly count from 1 to 10. Now, very quickly 1, 2, 3 . . . 4, 5, 6 . . . 7, 8, 9, and 10. Becoming energized like a bulb lighting up. Feel your body becoming energized, alert, active, and focused.

Now, I would like to offer some suggestions concerning your former depressive feelings. You were depressed early because you were condemning yourself, others, and the world. Where is it written that things must go the way you demand that they go? If you change your commands, demands, shoulds, oughts into preferences and wishes, you cannot feel extremely depressed. Actually, you will find that sadness is your alternative to depression.

Your automatic thoughts, many of which are irrational, dysfunctional, foolish, illogical, and crazy, have caused your former feelings of depression. Notice any foolish thoughts you may have had and then challenge those thoughts and replace them with more sensible thoughts such as "I can handle loss," "I can control my emotions," "I do not have to become or remain depressed," and "I can substitute sadness and remorse for depression."

In a few moments we will end this process, but before it ends you will remember, very deeply within your mind, what we have discussed. You will notice differences in your levels of depression. You will learn to control your emotions with your mind. Each day you will schedule activities. You will plan out your day and you will remain active daily. Each day you will become and remain more and more energized, more positive, optimistic, and you will believe in your future. You will find that your future is very important, and it will change as your thoughts and feelings change. Now, end this process by telling yourself that you can become dehypnotized. It is up to you at your own pace and rate.

Debriefing

It is important to determine how alert your client felt. Adjustments may have to be made to provide your client with the most active-alert suggestions. The next transcript deals with smoking cessation.

SMOKING

It is important not to hypnotize your client while he or she smokes, and it is important to contract with your client that hypnosis will only be used while he or she is not smoking. I find that it is important to discuss with my clients the health dangers of smoking, and I point out that weight gain can be associated with smoking cessation, but hypnosis can also be used to control weight gain. The following is the smoking cessation transcript.

Smoking Cessation Transcript

We will only use hypnosis when you are not smoking. Hypnosis will help you continue to be a nonsmoker. Close your eyes and let yourself relax. Yes, let your head, face, chest, stomach, and legs relax.

The dangers of smoking are well established. Smoking is one of the leading causes of death, and secondhand smoke is linked to lung cancer in nonsmoking people. You may not totally understand why you smoke, but smoking is a learned behavior. It is an addictive behavior.

You will learn to recognize the triggers of your smoking, such as wanting to smoke in the morning or after meals. Sometimes watching television stimulates the desire to smoke. You will recognize your triggers to smoke.

You can cope with your urges to smoke. First, exercising, deep breathing, chewing sugarless gum are some of the ways of handling your urge to smoke.

Your brain will search for substitutions to smoking. You will find strategies to cope with your smoking urges. When you get the urge to smoke, you will acknowledge it and say, "No!" You will say to yourself, "I am a nonsmoker and I do not have to smoke." Self-hypnosis or your ability to produce hypnosis outside of my office will serve as another coping strategy. Every day you will find a greater strength to maintain your nonsmoking status. Each day you do not smoke, you will get stronger and stronger.

Because you are a nonsmoker, you will not gain weight. You will find that you can control your appetite, just like the way you have learned to stop smoking. You will watch the fat and calories in your diet. You will have a desire to exercise and each and every day you will feel healthier and healthier.

Now, let's bring this process to an end. Slowly dehypnotize yourself, and as you are doing that, all the suggestions that I have given you will be processed deeply within your mind. It is up to you at your own pace and rate.

Debriefing

Clients have to receive encouragement to continue as nonsmokers and they need to remember that self-hypnosis and other coping techniques can help keep them to stay within the nonsmoking category. The next transcript deals with weight loss.

HYPNOSIS AND WEIGHT LOSS

Green (1999) and Levitt (1993) reported the effectiveness of hypnosis in treating obesity. When I use hypnosis for weight loss, I find that it is useful to work along with my client's physician. Hypnotic suggestions are similar to the ones for other habit disorders, such as smoking. The transcript that follows covers suggestions I have used to successfully help clients lose weight.

Hypnosis and Weight Loss Transcript

We are going to use hypnosis to help you lose weight. Now you get into a relaxed position and close your eyes. Let your body relax. You can start with your head, neck, back, trunk, legs, and feet. Your entire body is relaxing. Perhaps slowly or maybe quickly, but you are relaxing and letting tension go.

The thing to concern yourself with when using hypnosis for weight loss is your diet. Weight loss occurs when your caloric consumption decreases. Your short-term weight-loss goal should be between one to three pounds a week. High-bulk, low-calorie foods are the building blocks of an important diet which, of course, must become a way of life. Another thing you will find yourself doing is using a diet journal. That is, you will monitor your caloric intake. Also, you will remember to eat very slowly so that the hypothalamus of your brain can register fullness.

You will change your eating situation by eating at prescribed times in a certain room and following a certain ritual that will help you reduce your caloric intake. The last important factor of your weight loss program is exercise. You will need to exercise at least two to three times per week for at least 30 minutes.

As you starting losing weight, you will feel better about yourself, and you will be able to elicit self-hypnosis, which will allow you to manage cravings and hunger. Remember when you make a mistake during your weight loss plan, just recover and start over again.

Now it is time to dehypnotize yourself. It is up to you at your own rate and pace. Everything that we have discussed will be processed deeply within your own mind. Dehypnotize yourself now.

Debriefing

Process your client's reactions to the induction. Discuss possible modifications to the induction. The next transcript describes how to use hypnosis within the rehabilitation process.

HYPNOSIS AND REHABILITATION

Sapp, Farrell, Johnson, Sartin-Kirby, and Pumphrey (1997) described how rehabilitation counselors can apply hypnosis. It can be useful for helping clients recover from a disability, and it can be used to reduce stress related to returning to work. Using a repeated measures experimental design, Sapp (1995) found that relaxation therapy combined with hypnosis was effective in reducing anxiety and stress and in improving self-esteem of clients with neurogenic impairment. And four-week follow-up data found that treatment gains were maintained. Essentially, Sapp showed that hypnosis can decrease anxiety and strengthen self-esteem with clients who have experienced a disability.

Rehabilitation Hypnosis Transcript

Get into a relaxed position and close your eyes. Hypnosis can be used to help with your rehabilitation. First, you are more than your disability. Second, your disability is not related to your self-worth as a human being. Third, daily you will find yourself feeling stronger and stronger, not focusing on your disability. Fourth, daily, you will find yourself feeling happier, more content, more focused on rehabilitation, so that you start understanding your purpose in life. You will become very interested in understanding your purpose in life.

Let's talk a little about your thoughts concerning your disability. Many of your thoughts are based on your perception of social situations. Perhaps it is not the social situations that are producing some of your thoughts, but maybe they are mostly the byproducts of how you perceive things.

You must learn to have patience with your rehabilitation process. And you need to discern people for who they are, without judging them. When you are calm and patient, it becomes difficult to hurt people with your words or actions. You have to stop feeling hurt about things people say to you that are meant to be hurtful. Actually, criticism will roll off your back like water falling off the back of a duck. Hypnosis will give you the courage to take the "t" out of **can't** and find out that you can. If you want positive things to happen, you have to expect them to happen.

Yes, every day you will feel that life has a purpose, and you will have feelings of well-being. You are going to have feelings of personal safety, security, which you may not have felt in a long time. Each day you will become and remain more and more relaxed, both mentally and physically. All of these things are going to happen, just as I say they will. Of course, you are going to feel happier, content, cheerful, optimistic, less easily discouraged, and less easily depressed.

Now it is time to start dehypnotizing yourself. Whenever you go to sleep, you will get a restful sleep. Now slowly dehypnotize yourself. It is at your own rate and pace.

Debriefing

Discuss with your client his or her reaction to hypnosis. Clinically, I have found it useful to give clients, who are recovering from a disability, a taped recording of the hypnotic session.

POSSIBLE NEGATIVE SEQUELAE OF HYPNOSIS

Any form of psychotherapy can put a client at risk. For example, action strategies, psychotherapeutic procedures designed to move a client toward change, can pose risks for clients. Clinically, clients are particularly at risk when cognitive-behavioral or gestalt techniques are used, especially when these techniques are combined with hypnosis (Adrian 1996; Barber 1998; Sapp 1996).

The most probable negative sequelae of hypnosis, often overlooked by therapists, are transference and countertransference. Clinicians are aware that transference happens when a client projects feelings associated with significant others from the past onto the therapist. In contrast, countertransference occurs when a therapist attributes emotions and reactions from his or her past onto the client. Countertransference can make it difficult to manage therapeutic boundaries during hypnosis. For example, a therapist must be able to manage sexual feelings toward clients, especially ones stimulated by hypnosis. The literature clearly shows that countertransference is the leading contributor to the high rates of sexual involvement between therapists and clients (Adrian 1996; Sapp 1996).

Apparently, hypnosis can accelerate and intensify transference and countertransference, and therapists have to be prepared to handle these issues. The literature also suggests that therapists with narcissistic, antisocial, and power tendencies are more likely to engage in sexual relations with clients (Adrian 1995). If a therapist experiences sexual feelings toward a client as a result of hypnosis, it is imperative to comprehend such emotions and not to terminate prematurely hypnosis. Moreover, it is important to assert mentally and verbally the boundaries of the hypnotic relationship. And, finally, seek consultation.

Although seldom mentioned, as a result of hypnosis, clients can experience lethargy, confusion, anxiety, nausea, headaches, feelings of drowsiness, and nervousness (Barber 1998; Sapp 1996). Moreover, hypnosis can have prolongation effects; that is, hypnotic effects can continue after hypnosis has been terminated. For example, some clients have difficulty dehypnotizing, or they experience disorientation after hypnosis has ended (Barber 1998). Furthermore, therapists should use caution and have the clinical background when using hypnosis with clients experiencing psychosis, dissociative identity disorder, borderline personality disorder, posttraumatic stress disorder, and other severe disorders. It is important to stress constantly for therapists to use hypnosis to treat disorders that they have the training and skills to handle.

Some other possible negative sequelae of hypnosis are failures to cancel posthypnotic suggestions, dangers of masking illnesses, dangers of causing regressions, and the use of age progression techniques.

Finally, negative sequelae to hypnosis are infrequent, but therapists should alert themselves to the subtle forms of transference and countertransference that can occur as the result of hypnosis. Moreover, therapists should not be involved with the amateur use or stage uses of hypnosis, because it is unethical for an unqualified person to use hypnosis or to be instructed in the clinical uses of hypnosis. Hypnosis, when practiced by qualified practitioners, is relatively harmless and seldom will anything alarming occur; however, like any treatment that has a high effect size, hypnosis can produce harmful effects and beneficial ones. Even with appropriate termination procedures, hypnosis can lead to an alteration in information processing, and therapists need to be aware of possible negative after-effects of hypnosis.

CHAPTER CONCLUSION

This chapter emphasized treatment, and the minimum qualifications for using hypnosis is for a clinician to hold a master's degree in psychology, social work, mental health counseling, nursing, marriage and family therapy, or a related area. The major societies of hypnosis, the American Society of Clinical Hypnosis (ASCH), the Society for Clinical and Experimental Hypnosis (SCEH), and the International Society of Hypnosis (ISH) endorse the ethical uses of hypnosis. Specifically, clinicians who are not qualified to use hypnosis should not do so if they lack supervised clinical experience.

ASCH, a clinical society, is the largest hypnosis society in the United States. It offers annual workshops and provides certification in clinical hypnosis. Also, SCEH, a relatively small research-oriented society, offers scientific meetings and annual workshops. Finally, ISH is an international society that includes members from both ASCH and SCEH. Like ASCH and SCEH, ISH offers workshops and scientific meetings. Clinicians can contact ASCH at (312) 645-9810; SCEH at (509) 332-7555; and ISH at (011) 61-3-9496-4105.

Chapter 6

CONTEMPORARY HYPNOSIS THEORIES AND RESEARCH

CHAPTER OVERVIEW

THIS CHAPTER DESCRIBES contemporary hypnosis theories and research. First, Barber's, Spanos', and Hilgard's theories are described. Second, Barber's 3-dimensional paradigm is described. Third, a summary and conclusion for research is presented. Fourth, measures of hypnotic responding are described. Fifth, hypnosis and memory are discussed. Sixth, instruments for hypnotic depth, vividness of imagination, and dissociation are described. Finally, hypnosis, automaticity, involuntariness, and nonvolitional responding are described along with a critique of Kirsch and Lynn's new sociocognitive theory of hypnotic involuntariness.

CONTEMPORARY HYPNOSIS THEORIES AND RESEARCH

Theodore Sarbin in the 1950s was one of the first theorists to reject the altered state notion of hypnosis, and he viewed hypnosis as social psychological behavior. More specifically, he viewed hypnosis as a form of role taking, not role playing, because role playing suggests a sham and dissembling behavior.

Sarbin conceptualized hypnosis as a dramaturgical metaphor and he used role theory to explain the automaticity of hypnotic experiences. Furthermore, Sarbin was aware that hypnosis altered clients' subjective perceptions, and he recognized individual differences in hypnotic responsiveness (Barber 1999).

Barber's Paradigm

Theodore X. Barber (1969) was the second major theorist to reject the altered-state conceptualization of hypnosis. Barber did intense experimentation on hypnosis using an inductive approach, and he found that several variables affected hypnotic responsiveness. For example, the clients' attitudes, their expectancies, the wording of the situation as hypnosis, the wording and the tone of suggestions, clients' motivation, the wording of the inquiry, and the behavior of the hypnotist all affect hypnotic responsiveness.

Barber rejected the trance concept because he found from study after study that hypnosis could be elicited without a hypnotic induction. He found that increased hypnotic suggestibility could be produced by increasing the client's motivation and expectancy. Curiously, absent from Barber's theory are any stable personality traits.

As stated previously, absorption, fantasy proneness, and dissociation are reliably related to hypnotic suggestibility, but they account for about one percent of the variance. Although the attitudes of the client and expectancies account for more variance, most of the variance that explains hypnotic suggestibility remains unaccounted for (Barber 1999). This is what makes hypnotic suggestibility a curious concept, because test-retest reliabilities of hypnotic suggestibility scales calculated after several intervals over a 25-year period rival those of intelligence tests (Piccione, Hilgard & Zimbardo 1989).

Spanos

Spanos (1986, 1996) stressed the importance of goal-directed fantasies as a mechanism for generating hypnotic involuntariness. He conceptualized hypnotic responding as a strategic role enactment geared toward the client convincing himself or herself and others that he or she is experiencing hypnosis or the suggested state of affairs.

Hilgard

Barber (1999) argued that Hilgard (1965) started with a strong altered-state theory of hypnosis and later Hilgard and Hilgard (1975) weakened his state concept to imply that the altered-state notion of hypnosis is a descriptive label and it does not imply causation. It appears that Hilgard used the term "trance" to describe clients' subjective experiences during hypnosis. Recently, Hilgard (1991, 1994) presented dissociation as the explanatory mechanism of hypnosis. Even more recently, Woody and Bowers (1994) presented another altered-state theory of hypnosis, referred to as dissociated control theory. This theory suggests that hypnosis weakens the executive control of behavior in a way that parallels clients with frontal lobe damage. Because hypnosis weakens frontal lobe brain control, suggestions by the hypnotist can activate responses directly; however, this theory has difficulty explaining self-hypnosis.

Barber's 3-Dimensional Paradigm

Barber proposed that there are three hypnotic types of clients—the fantasy-prone, amnesic-prone, and positively-set.

Fantasy-Prone

Wilson and Barber (1981/1983) interviewed 27 women, mostly professionals, who were selected from a large group of excellent hypnotic subjects. These women had the following commonalities in their backgrounds: a long history of make-believe and fantasy, vivid memories dating back to the age of 3, and ability to use their minds to affect their bodies. To illustrate, many of these women were able to experience pseudocyesis, false pregnancy, which led to the cessation of their menstrual cycles, bloating stomach, morning sickness, and the craving for certain foods. Finally, many of these women reported paranormal or psychic experiences, such as during childhood, in which they lived in make-believe worlds. For example, during childhood they thought that their dolls were alive; they believed in angels, fairies, and other supernatural beings.

Many of these women were encouraged to develop their fantasies by significant others and they used their fantasies to escape from lonely existences. Moreover, training in ballet, drama, and other skills involving these women's imaginations stimulated their fantasy development.

The Amnesic-Prone

Barrett (1990, 1996) studied 34 highly hypnotic subjects from a population of 1200 participants. She found that certain participants had amnesia for hypnosis. In addition, certain subjects were amnesic during their daily lives. Actually, 60 percent of these subjects had spontaneous amnesia for hypnotic events. Moreover, all subjects showed consistent and total posthypnotic amnesia when it was suggested. Barrett did not find spontaneous amnesia with her fantasy-prone subjects. When amnesia was suggested to her fantasy-prone subjects, one-third failed the item and two-thirds had partial recall or knew they could counter the suggestion.

Barrett's study found marked differences between fantasy-prone and amnesic-prone participants when they were dehypnotized. For example, the fantasy-prone subjects exhibited a smile when they dehypnotized, while the amnesic-prone dehypnotized subject felt confused and they attributed their experiences to the skills of hypnosis. In contrast, the fantasy-prone subjects attributed their responses to their imaginations.

In terms of hallucinations, there were differences between the two groups of subjects. Specifically, the fantasy-prone subjects knew that they had produced the hallucinations and they remembered the hypnotist's suggestions for hallucinations. In contrast, the amnesic-prone could not remember the hypnotist's suggestions for hallucinations and believed typically that their hallucinations were real.

Interestingly, the amnesic-prone subjects exhibited general forgetfulness in their lives and most had no memory before the age of 5. Forty percent could not remember life events before the ages of 6 and 8. In a striking contrast, all of Barrett's fantasy-prone individuals had vivid memories before the age of 3 and most had memories before the age of 2. Another striking characteristic of the amnesic-prone were their reports of having been beaten, battered, injured, and suffered psychological abuse or sexual abuse during childhood.

Curiously, amnesic-prone were not fantasy-prone, and the amnesic-prone reported mundane and narrow fantasies about their future. Moreover, the amnesic-prone could become absorbed in fantasies of others through books, plays, and so on. Essentially, these amnesic-prone subjects' imaginations had an external locus of control, and Barrett referred to them as dissociators.

To summarize, the amnesic-prone differed from the fantasy-prone in that they needed an extensive hypnotic induction and they experienced a loss of muscle tone, exhibited a very subdued voice, and had lethargic movements. In contrast to the fantasy-prone, the amnesic-prone did not report psychic experiences like ghosts, telepathy, and out-of-body experiences.

The Positively-Set Clients

These individual have positive attitudes toward hypnosis and toward the clinician employing hypnosis. Moreover, these clients have positive motivations to perform well on the experiences suggested and they have positive expectancies. Furthermore, these individuals are able to think with or imagine the suggested phenomena. Herbert Spiegel and Connery (1982) described these clients as conforming, trusting, and imaginative. Other researchers, such as Spanos (1991), Kirsch (1991), Wagstaff (1991), Sarbin (1999), Coe and Sarbin (1991), Lynn and Rhue (1991), Sheehan and McConkey (1982) made similar conclusions. Finally, Pekala, Kumar, and Marcano's (1995) cluster analysis research supported these three hypnotic types of subjects.

Summary and Conclusions for Research

Barber (1999) argues that the "trance" view of hypnosis more or less describes the hypnotic responsiveness of many amnesic-prone subjects, and the "nonstate" position describes the behavior of many positively-set subjects. Barber concludes that neither view, state nor nonstate, describes the behavior of the fantasy-prone subject. In terms of research, Barber's new paradigm suggests that hypnotizability and the three types of subjects should be studied within factorial designs. Specifically, hypnotizability and the three types of subjects may interact in complex ways. Finally, the following 3 X 3 factorial design would allow a researcher to study some of these complex interactions and main effects:

Types of Subjects

		1	2	3
	High			
Hypnotizability	Medium			
	Low			

3 X 3 Factorial Design

Sapp (1999, Chapter 4) describes factorial designs as multiple-treatment designs in which there are more than one independent variable. Sapp (1997b, Chapter 2, 1999, Chapter 1) defined independent variables as classification variables such as types of subjects (fantasy-prone, amnesic-prone, and positively-set) and hypnotizability (high, medium, and low). It is apparent that the types of subjects variable has three levels (subcategories) and that hypnotizability has three levels; if we combined types of subjects and hypnotizability into the same experiment, we will have a 3 X 3 factorial design. It is worth noting, that within psychotherapy, treatments are referred to as independent variables; therefore, any treatment can be regarded as an independent variable. The purpose of factorial designs is to investigate the interactional effects of two independent variables on some measurement(s) or dependent variable(s).

If the types of subjects interacted with hypnotizability, this suggests that simultaneously both variables have an effect on some dependent variable(s), and the results are not due to a single independent variable (main effect).

In addition to Barber's three-dimensional paradigm, he recommends that researchers investigate three other dimensions. First of these is the social-psychological dimension or experiences associated with being a participant in a hypnosis experiment such as demand characteristics or the subtle cues that subjects detect from an experiment that provide clues to the purpose of the study. Moreover, expectancies, social roles, and rules affect participants' behavior within experiments.

Second, the hypnotist dimension pivots on the fact that hypnosis is a complex social interplay between a client and therapist. And all the factors that affect general psychotherapy such as empathy, genuineness, and so on, also impact the types of subjects and hypnotizability.

The third dimension is the kinds of suggestions used. For example, hypnotic suggestions can be direct or authoritative or indirect or permissive (i.e., Ericksonian hypnosis). Moreover, hypnotic suggestions can involve imagery, dissociation, regression, and so on.

To summarize, Barber's new paradigm does explain why there has been contention between special process and nonstate theorists. The contention appears to be due to the fact that each group of researchers never saw all three types of subjects (fantasy-prone, amnesic-prone, and positively-set). Barber's new paradigm helps unify the disagreement between state and nonstate theories; however, it remains to be seen if new brain imagining techniques will detect individual differences in brain functioning with a client undergoing hypnosis (Zahn, Moraga & Ray 1996). Nevertheless, brain correlates of differences in clients undergoing hypnosis are not sufficient proof that hypnosis is an altered state of consciousness. The varied experimental evidence does not support the belief that hypnosis is an altered state of consciousness. Finally, hypnosis appears to be a sociocognitive phenomenon in which clients can alter their subjective experiences and hypnosis can be explained without reifying the special process construct.

MEASURES OF HYPNOTIC RESPONDING

Hypnotic responsiveness refers to the individual differences that a client or subject shows to hypnosis, and it exists on a continuum. Correlates of hypnotic responsiveness include, but are not limited to, ideomotor and ideosensory responding; cognitive abilities such as imagery, fantasy-proneness, and absorption; sensory denial or negation such as analgesia or negative hallucinations; perceptual distortions such as positive hallucinations and hyperesthesia; and posthypnotic suggestions such as amnesia and dissociation.

Hypnotizability scales are standardized measures that determine the level of responsiveness a client or subject has to hypnosis (Council 1999; Kirsch 1997; Sapp 1997d). Kirsch differentiates between hypnotizability, the increase in suggestibility following a hypnotic induction, and suggestibility, a construct that does not require an induction. Furthermore, Kirsch pointed out that a minority of clients or subjects do not report an increase in suggestibility following a hypnotic induction.

Piccone, Hilgard, and Zimbardo (1989) noted that many hypnotizability scales rest on the assumption that hypnotizability is a **stable trait**. Even though hypnotizability appears to be a stable trait, it is also affected by the client's or subject's expectations and social psychological factors. Lastly, many hypnotizability scales are based on the classic suggestion effect, the subjective experience clients or subjects have that their hypnotic responses are automatic (Sapp 1997a).

Many clinicians and researchers confuse hypnotic susceptibility with **hypnotic depth**. A client's hypnotic depth is his or her subjective experience of low, medium, or deep levels of hypnosis. Clinically, a client can score highly on a hypnotizability scale but may not experience deep levels of hypnosis. The following scale has been used in hypnosis research to measure hypnotic depth (Sapp & Evanow 1998).

HYPNOTIC DEPTH

I would like to know the depth of your hypnotic experience. Please circle a number between 0 and 10 that best indicates the depth of hypnosis you experienced.

0	"I did not experience hypnosis" (wide awake—no perceptual alterations).
1	
2	"I had a slight experience of hypnosis."
3	
4	
5	"I felt a moderate level of hypnosis."
6	
7	"I felt a deep level of hypnosis."
8	
9	
10	"I felt the deepest possible level of hypnosis."

If a client endorses zero, this suggests that he or she did not experience hypnosis. A score of 5 indicates medium depth, and a score of 10 suggests the deepest level of hypnosis.

The Stanford Scale of Hypnotic Susceptibility (SHSS), Forms A, B, and C are the benchmarks for individual measures of hypnotic susceptibility (Weitzenhoffer & Hilgard 1959, 1967). These scales start with an induction, and they are representative of hypnotic experiences. Forms A and B have a reliability measure of .83, and the required time for testing is about 50 minutes. And Form C has a reliability measure of .85; it samples fantasy and cognitive distortion better than Forms A and B. Form C has the following items: hand lowering, moving hands apart, mosquito hallucination, taste hallucination, arm rigidity, dream, age regression, arm immobilization, anosmia to ammonia, voice hallucination, negative visual hallucination, and posthypnotic amnesia. The Stanford Scales are scored on an objective criteria ranging between zero and 12. If a client did not respond to any items, he or she would receive a score of zero, and if a client responded to all items, he or she would obtain a score of 12.

Approximately the same time the Stanford Scales were being developed during the 1950s and early 1960s, the Harvard Group Scale of Hypnotic Susceptibility, Form A (HGSHS:A, Shor & Orne, 1962). The HGSHS:A was derived from the Stanford Scales, and it is the benchmark standard for group measures of hypnotizability. The HGSHS:A is a 12-item scale that has a reliability measure of .83, and it contains the following items: head falling, hand lowering, arm immobilization, finger lock, arm rigidity, hands moving together, verbal inhibition, communication inhibition, hallucination of a fly, eye catalepsy, posthypnotic suggestion, and posthypnotic amnesia. It takes about an hour to administer this scale.

Bowers (1993, 1998) has published another group scale in its entirety in the *International Journal of Clinical and Experimental Hypnosis* called the Waterloo-Stanford Group Scale of Hypnotic Susceptibility, Form C (WSGS). This scale is an adaptation of the SHSS:C. The WSGS has a reliability measure of .80, and it consists of 12 items and scores can range from 0 to 12.

Another Stanford scale, the Stanford Hypnotic Clinical Scale (SHCS) is a brief scale that requires about 20 minutes to administer. This is a clinical scale that correlates .72 with the SHSC:C (Hilgard & Hilgard 1975).

A scale that provides a profile of hypnotic abilities is the Stanford Profile Scale of Hypnotic Ability, Forms I and II (SPS:I&II). These scales explore the limits of hypnotic ability; they do not provide a single score (Weitzenhoffer & Hilgard 1959, 1967).

The Hypnotic Induction Profile (HIP; Spiegel & Spiegel 1978) is yet another brief clinical scale that requires about 10 minutes to administer. The HIP has a reliability measure of .76, but its correlations with the SHSS:A are between .22 and .32. The most controversial aspect of this scale is the "eye roll" test, which Spiegel and Spiegel refer to as a hypothetical physiological indicator of hypnotizability. The eye roll score is based on the client rolling his or her eyes upward. This item is scored based on the amount of sclera visible. The validity of the HIP is questionable, and the research findings that correlate the HIP with other hypnotizability measures are mixed (Council 1999; Perry et al. 1992; Sheehan & McConkey 1982).

There are Stanford scales that have been adapted for use with children and adolescents. The Children's Hypnotic Susceptibility Scale (CHSS) was adapted from the SHSS:A and B and the SPS:I and II. The CHSS has two parts; Part I is for children (ages 5 through 12 years) and Part II is for adolescents (age 13 through 16 years) (London 1962).

The Stanford Hypnotic Clinical Scale for Children (SHCSC, Forms A and B), the adult version, is a brief clinical scale. Form B of this scale correlates .67 with an adaptation of the SHSS:A for children (Council 1999).

HYPNOTIZABILITY SCALES REFLECTING A COGNITIVE-BEHAVIORAL ORIENTATION

The Stanford scales reflect a traditional approach to hypnosis that relies on classic hypnotic phenomena, and these scales rely on sleep suggestions, direct suggestions, and a trance induction. In contrast to the Stanford Scales, the Barber Suggestibility Scale

(BSS) (Barber 1969), the Creative Imagination Scale (CIS) (Barber & Wilson 1979; Wilson & Barber 1981, 1983), and the Carleton University Responsiveness to Suggestion Scale (CURSS) (Spanos, Radtke, Hodgins, Stam & Bertrand 1983), reflect a cognitive-behavioral approach to hypnotizability (Council 1999).

Both the BSS and CIS can be given without an induction. The BSS contains the following eight items: arm lowering, arm levitation, hand lock, thirst hallucination, verbal inhibition, body immobility, posthypnotic-like response, and selective amnesia. Scores on the BSS range between 0 and 24, and it has a reliability measure between .80 and .88. Barber and Wilson (1979) and Sapp (1997a; 1997d) pointed out that the major difficulty of this scale is its authoritarian nature.

As a response to the authoritarian nature and directedness of the BSS, the CIS was developed. It can be administered in groups or individually and can be used for clinical and experimental purposes. Although the CIS can be used with a hypnotic induction, it does not contain one; it uses guided imagination instructions to facilitate clients' abilities to experience the suggested effects. The following are the 10 items on the CIS: arm heaviness, hand levitation, finger anesthesia, water hallucination, olfactory-gustatory hallucination, music hallucination, temperature hallucination, time distortion, age regression, and mind-body relaxation. After the last suggestion, clients self-score their responses to the suggested effects. Scores range between 0 and 40. In terms of psychometric properties, the CIS has a reliability measure of .82, and it correlates significantly with the BSS, HGSHS, Form A, and SHSS:C. In summary, both the BSS and CIS are briefer scales than the Stanford scales and HGSHS, Form A. Finally, the CIS is especially useful for clients who fear losing control or for clients who fear hypnosis.

The CURSS is methodologically similar to the BSS, just like the HGSHS:A is similar to the SHSS:A. The CURSS takes less than 15 minutes to administer and can be administered to individuals or groups. The CURSS contains the following seven test suggestions: arm rising, arms moving apart, arm catalepsy, arm immobility, auditory hallucination, visual hallucination, and amnesia. Very similar to the HGSHS:A, the CURSS is self-scored by the client. Like the BSS, the CURSS has an objective and subjective scoring system. In addition, the CURSS has an objective involuntariness scale that consists of behaviorally passing items and experiencing them as occurring involuntarily. In terms of factor structure, the CURSS has a factor structure that is similar to the SHSS:C, and it correlates .65 with the SHSS:C. Finally, the BSS, CIS, and CURSS are brief cognitive-behavioral approaches to hypnotizability.

INDIRECT HYPNOTIC SUSCEPTIBILITY SCALE

Clinicians and researchers who follow the Ericksonian tradition to hypnosis will find the Wexler-Alman Indirect Hypnotic Susceptibility Scale (WAIHSS), which is an adaptation of the SHSS:A and the HGSHS:A, useful for individual or group administration. The WAIHSS is an indirect hypnotic susceptibility scale that contains 12 items. This scale is available from Brian M. Alman, 3430 Camino Del Rio, N., Suite 104, San Diego, CA 92108.

HYPNOTIZABILITY MEASURES AND THEORETICAL PERSPECTIVES

The Stanford scales and Harvard scale are connected to the traditional perspective of hypnosis. In contrast, the BSS, CIS, and CURSS are associated with the cognitive-behavioral perspective of hypnosis. Lastly, the Wexler-Alman scale was developed to tap into the Ericksonian perspective of hypnosis.

HYPNOSIS AND MEMORY

Memory is a reconstruction process based on the context that one happens to be in. For example, memory does not work like a tape recorder, and memory is easily distorted by one's expectations, mood states, and information obtained after the original experience (Spanos 1996). Mandler (1984) and Neisser (1976) have found that expectations can distort and facilitate memory.

For example, Brewster and Treyens (1981) had subjects wait in an office of a graduate student presumably for an experimenter. Later, subjects were taken to a different room and were asked to describe the graduate student's office. Many subjects reported seeing books in the graduate student's office, but there were not any books in the office. Subjects had the expectations that an academic office would contain books. This study highlights how people can hold implicit, yet erroneous, expectations. Also, this study illustrates how memory is restructured based upon a social context (Loftus 1979, 1993; Yant 1992).

Some therapists assume that postevent information and a client's confidence in his or her recall are indicative of an accurate memory. Postevent information, or information given retrospectively about a memory, can lead to distortions (Yant 1992). Moreover, Bothwell and Deffenbacher (1987), Wells (1993), and Wells and Murray (1984) found that the relationship between accuracy of recall and confidence in recall is statistically nonsignificant (Spanos 1996).

Finally, Neisser (1989) and Neisser and Harsh (1992) found that even when subjects experience very salient and frightening events, their memories can be altered and distorted with the passage of time. In summary, memory is a reconstructive process that can be influenced by many variables such as the passage of time, expectations, the social context, and so on. There is no experimental evidence to support the use of hypnosis to refresh memory. Spanos (1996) reported that hypnosis can increase false as well as accurate memories, and a clinician has difficulty in determining if a memory is accurate; therefore, this clinician does not recommend hypnosis as a technique to enhance memory.

HYPNOSIS, AUTOMATICITY, INVOLUNTARINESS, AND NONVOLITIONAL RESPONDING

Not only is hypnosis an adjunctive procedure to psychotherapy or medicine in which one person (therapist) offers to another person (terms the client) suggestions that can produce psychophysiological changes, but hypnosis and other complex behaviors are automatic, nonvolitional, and volitional, especially at the point of intention. Bargh and Barndollar (1996) described the following four necessary conditions for a behavioral action to be automatic:
1. The behavioral action is outside of awareness.
2. The behavioral action cannot be prevented; hence, it is uncontrollable and unstoppable.
3. The behavioral action does not require volitional effort; hence it is unintentional or nonvolitional.
4. The behavioral action does not require attentional resources.

Each of these conditions leads to a series of complicated issues. First, ideomotor and ideosensory theorists assume that hypnotic responding is automatic; nevertheless, as Kirsch and Lynn (1997), Woody and Farvolden (1998), Spiegel (1998), and Hilgard (1991, 1994) noted, the volitional status of hypnotic responding is an extremely debated topic. Three theories, neodissociation, dissociated control, and sociocognitive, offer different reasons for why clients report that their responses to hypnotic suggestions feel involuntary.

Hilgard (1991, 1994), a proponent of the neodissociation theory, explains automatic hypnotic responding using dissociation as the mechanism. Before Hilgard, Jean Marie Charcot (1825–1893) and his student, Pierre Janet (1859–1947), described a dissociation theory of hypnotic responding. According to their theory, a client who has been exposed to psychological stress or trauma is more likely to experience dissociation, or the separation of ideas and behavioral patterns that are normally associated.

Hilgard's (1991, 1994) theory differs from Charcot's and Janet's in that his theory of dissociation is one of an incomplete dissociation among cognitive systems. According to this theory, automatic hypnotic responding is the result of dissociation among an executive ego, a central processing unit that monitors activities, and cognitive subsystems. Moreover, Hilgard proposed that a combination of dissociation and the client's ability to erect an amnesic barrier among dissociated parts explains how hypnotic responding occurs.

Dissociated control theory, as proposed by Woody and Farvolden (1998), is also a dissociation theory of automatic hypnotic responding, but this theory questioned the amnesic barrier notion of the neodissociation theory. This theory hypothesizes that hypnosis weakens or inhibits frontal lobe functioning in much the same way as a client with frontal lobe damage. Curiously, this theory cannot explain self-hypnosis, because it states that a clinician must externally activate hypnotic schemata within a client, and this theory requires a special state or condition (altered state of consciousness). Finally, the dissociated control theory views clients who elicit hypnosis as being similar to clients with frontal lobe disorders. In summary, both the neodissociation and dissociated control theories view hypnosis as the result of dissociation and an alteration in a client's conscious functioning. Finally, these theories are viewed as special processes, or theories that propose that hypnosis results in an altered state of consciousness that differs from normal consciousness.

Spanos (1986, 1991) proposed a sociocognitive theory of hypnotic responding. In fact, Spanos viewed hypnotic responding as intentional rather than automatic, and he believed that clients convince themselves that their intentional responses are automatic. Oddly, Spanos stated that clients are unaware of their intentions, and this is what makes clients believe that their responses to hypnotic suggestions are automatic; clients make errors of misattribution. But how do clients misattribute the causes of their hypnotic responses? Recently, Kirsh and Lynn (1997, 1999) proposed a new sociocognitive theory or response set theory of hypnotic involuntariness.

Kirsch and Lynn (1997, 1998a,b, 1999) were influenced by several social and cognitive theorists (Bargh 1994; Bargh & Barndollar 1996; Bargh & Gollwitzer 1994; Dixon, Brunet & Laurence 1990; Dixon & Laurence 1992; Lynn 1992; Lynn & Rhue 1994) and by Kirsch's (1990, 1997) theory of response expectancy (Page, Hanley & Green 1997). Kirsch and Lynn (1997, 1998a,b) argued that routinized behaviors are automatic. Moreover, therapies based on principles of classical conditioning, such as systematic desensitization, describe reactions as being automatic. For example, if a strong stream of air (unconditioned stimulus) is blown into one's face, one's automatic reaction is to blink (unconditioned response). Actually, Van Den Hout and Merkelbach (1991) argued that classical conditioning can be applied to involuntary and voluntary responses. Furthermore, Van Den Hout and Merkelbach presented a neo-Pavlovian theory of classical conditioning that states that clients anticipate the probability relationship among stimuli (Sapp 1997b). Finally, this neo-classical conditioning theory states that clients can respond to automatic and intentional responses.

Norman and Shallice (1986) further clarified this point by stating that all behavior is initiated automatically through interactive hierarchically arranged sensory motor schemata. Schemata theory explains how clients form beliefs, attitudes, attributions, and so on (Bartlett 1932; Granvold 1994; Piaget 1926). Moreover, schemata theory describes how clients discriminate attributional actions as involuntary and nonvolitional.

When one argues that hypnotic responding is nonvolitional this suggests that the experiences appear to happen automatically. Indeed, often clients report that their subjective responses and experiences with hypnosis occurred automatically. To say that a hypnotic experience is nonvolitional suggests that clients' subjective hypnotic experiences occur without conscious or volitional effort. The term involuntary has a connotation of being unpreventable, or occurring against the client's will (Kirsch 1990). Even though clients report their hypnotic experiences are nonvolitional, they are aware that they could terminate their experience at any point. Similar to Spanos, Sarbin (1998) theorizes that nonvolitional hypnotic responding is a post hoc inference that participants have about their behavior. Sarbin describes how the interaction between the clinician and client and contextual cues help the client and clinician define the environment in which hypnosis will be elicited (Fourie 1991).

Recently, ironic process theory has been applied to hypnotic responding and involuntary behavior (Wegner 1994; Wegner and Wheatley 1999). According to this theory, when a client attempts to control his or her mind, two opposing processes occur: an intentional operating process that searches for a desired state of mind and an ironic monitoring process that automatically searches for ways to not achieve the desired state.

Suppose, for example, that an alcoholic was attempting to abstain from drinking. The intentional operating process would search for thoughts that were consistent with not drinking; in contrast, the ironic monitoring process would search for counterproductive cognition related to drinking. Examples of ironic monitoring cognition could be, "drinking will relax you; drinking will give you a buzz." It is theorized that the ironic monitoring process is automatic; therefore, this theory has implications for hypnotic responding. The implication is that a client is actively preventing hypnotic responses from occurring as simple voluntary acts. For example, with arm immobilization, the intentional operating process may try to prevent voluntary arm immobilization, whereas the ironic monitoring process would search for thoughts that would produce arm immobilization. Theoretically, since ironic monitoring process is automatic, cognitive load should increase arm immobilization.

Recently, Kirsch and Lynn (1999) included ironic response set theory to their sociocognitive theory. And response set theory assumes that at the moment of activation, all behavior is initiated automatically. Hence, automaticity is the result of clients' judgments, intentions, situational cues, culturally derived knowledge and beliefs, response expectancies, and the consistency of their goals. Finally, according to this theory, cognitive load should inhibit responses to many suggestions. In conclusion, response set theory suggests that all behavior is initiated automatically, as opposed to conscious intentions. The next paragraph will describe how the brain is implicated in mental causation and clients' awareness of intentions.

Wegner and Wheatley (1999) and Libet (1985) found that brain activity preceded the onset of voluntary action. Specifically, Libet (1985) found using readiness potential (RP), a scalp-recorded slow negative shift in electrical potential, that RP began up to a second or more before voluntary motor acts. Moreover, Libet found that RP preceded movement, which was measured electromyographically, by at least 550 milliseconds. Furthermore, Libet asked participants to recall the position of a clock once they were initially aware of intending to move their fingers. Even when adjustments were made for the time it took participants to monitor a clock, participants' awareness of their intentions followed their RPs by 350–400 milliseconds.

In summary, even though participants' conscious intentions preceded their finger movements, they occurred after brain events. These results suggest that conscious intentions may not cause actions, but brain events may cause intentions and actions. Furthermore, Wegner and Wheatley (1999) presented a plausible argument that the sense that a client has intentionally caused an action is frequently an error; therefore, clients can mistakenly believe that they have intentionally caused an act when, in fact, they were forced to perform an act because they were led to think about the act just before it occurred. Finally, the model that follows, Norman and Shallice (1986), describes how behavior is initiated.

Norman and Shallice (1986) described a two-tier system that explains the initiation of behavior. Contention scheduling, the lower system, handles routine behavior and tasks, and the supervisory attentional system controls nonroutine actions (Woody & Farvolden 1998). Within Norman and Shallice's model, volition is associated with the supervisory system. Even though their model is similar to Hilgard's (1991, 1994) neodissociation theory of nonvolitional hypnotic responding, it does not require an amnesiac barrier or an altered state of consciousness. From a clinical standpoint, clients enter therapy with the intent and expectation that they will benefit from hypnosis; therefore, clients' responses to hypnosis are intentional and automatic, and clients enter therapy with the expectation that their responses will occur involuntarily.

Kirsch and Lynn (1997, 1998a,b, 1999) state that imaginative ability, fantasy proneness, and expectations bolster clients' perceptions of involuntariness. In contrast to the neodissociation and dissociated control theory, Kirsch and Lynn do not use a special condition resembling frontal lobe disorders or alterations in clients' consciousness to explain clients' automatic hypnotic responding. Moreover, Kirsch and Lynn's theory allows for self-hypnosis, and they describe how volitional and nonvolitional behavior can occur within and outside of hypnosis. Furthermore, they are aware that all complex behaviors are automatic and intentional.

Apparently, Kirsch and Lynn's (1997, 1998a,b, 1999) theory can account for more data in explaining automaticity than do the neodissociation and dissociated control theories; however, Bartis and Zamasky (1990) reported that clients could respond to hypnotic suggestions while they were visualizing conflicting scenes. Moreover, Bartis and Zamansky found that highly susceptible clients were able to experience hypnosis with and without imagery; therefore, imagery is not the sole mechanism of hypnotic responding.

There are several other issues with Kirsch and Lynn's (1997, 1998a,b, 1999) theory. First, it cannot adequately explain hypnotic analgesia. Specifically, Hargadon, Bowers, and Woody (1995) did not find that goal-directed suggestions versus suggestions without imagery enhanced analgesia. Another difficulty with this theory is it cannot adequately explain individual differences to hypnotic susceptibility. For example, Hilgard (1965) found that hypnotic susceptibility was normally distributed. If fantasy proneness, expectancies, goal-directed fantasies, and other sociocognitive factors accounted for most of the variance on hypnotic susceptibility measures, these measures would not be normally distributed.

This writer notes that Kirsch and Lynn (1997, 1998a,b, 1999) are correct when they say that imagery can enhance hypnotic responding, but hypnotic responding appears to have trait-like features (Piccone, Hilgard & Zimbardo 1989). Furthermore, this writer agrees with Kirsch and Lynn's position that hypnotic responsiveness is modifiable (Spanos 1986; Wickless and Kirsch 1989), but it is not indefinitely modifiable. Actually, it is impossible to turn clients who score low on hypnotic susceptibility measures into clients who are highly responsive to hypnosis. To summarize, dissociation, absorption, fantasy proneness, and expectancies are only some of the factors of automatic hypnotic responding. Finally, one theory cannot explain all of the features or the mechanisms of hypnosis, because hypnosis consists of many facets. Also, Pashler's (1998) theory of automaticity is not a fact, but hypnosis is a theory, and it is a fact of everyday life. In conclusion, evidence-based research will determine if theories of automaticity complement theories of hypnosis.

RESEARCH INSTRUMENTS

The following research instruments will be described: Vividness of Imagination Scale (VIS), Hypnosis Survey (HS), Description of Hypnotic Experience (DHE), Description of Hypnotic Regression Experience (DHRE), and General Dissociation Scale (GDS).

The VIS is used to get clients to rate their vividness of imagination. This scale is extremely useful for evaluating imagery-based inductions. A score of 0 indicates that the client did not experience vivid imagination, and a score of 10 indicates that a client experienced the most vivid imagination.

Name_____

Circle the item that corresponds to your experience.

Vividness Of Imagination Scale (VIS)

0   I did not experience any vivid imagination.

1

2   I slightly experienced vivid imagination.

3

4

5   I experienced a moderate level of vivid imagination.

6

7

    I experienced a large amount of vivid imagination.

8

9

10   I experienced the most vivid imagination possible.

The HS measures clients' misconceptions of hypnosis (Page, Handley, & Green, 1997).

Name_____

Circle the item that corresponds to your experience.

Hypnosis Survey (HS)

1.
Everyone can experience hypnosis.   Yes   No

If yes, to what extent?

(a little)   (very much)
1   2   3   4   5   6   7

2.
Hypnosis results in a loss of consciousness.   Yes   No
If yes, to what extent?

(a little)   (very much)
1   2   3   4   5   6   7

3.
Hypnosis weakens ones will.   Yes   No
If yes, to what extent?

(a little)   (very much)
1   2   3   4   5   6   7

4.
Hypnosis can cure physical ailments.   Yes   No
If yes, to what extent?

(a little)   (very much)
1   2   3   4   5   6   7

5.
Hypnosis can cure mental illnesses.   Yes   No
If yes, to what extent?

(a little)   (very much)
1   2   3   4   5   6   7

6.
To become hypnotized, one must be gullible and have a weak mind.   Yes   No
If yes, to what extent?

(a little) (very much)
1   2   3   4   5   6   7

7.
People can be hypnotized against their will.   Yes   No
If yes, to what extent?

(a little) (very much)
1   2   3   4   5   6   7

8.
Hypnosis can lead to demonic possession.   Yes   No
If yes, to what extent?

(a little) (very much)
1   2   3   4   5   6   7

9.
Most people cannot remember experiencing hypnosis.   Yes   No
If yes, to what extent?

(a little) (very much)
1   2   3   4   5   6   7

10.
Hypnosis is mind over matter—a mind game.   Yes   No
If yes, to what extent?
(a little) (very much)
1   2   3   4   5   6   7

11.
Do you think you can experience hypnosis?   Yes   No
If yes, to what extent?

(a little)   (very much)
1   2   3   4   5   6   7

The DHE measures whether a client has experienced absorption and/or hypnosis (Radtke & Spanos, 1982

Name_____

Description of Hypnotic Experience
(Adapted from Radtke and Spanos, 1982)

Circle the item that corresponds to your experience.
1. I was not hypnotized nor absorbed while responding to suggestions.
2. I experienced the effects of the suggestions. I was absorbed in the suggestions, and I was hypnotized while responding to a slight degree.
3. I experienced the effects of the suggestions. I was absorbed in the suggestions, and I was hypnotized while responding to a moderate degree.
4. I experienced the effects of the suggestions. I was absorbed in the suggestions, and I was hypnotized while responding to a high degree.
5. I experienced the effects of the suggestions. I was absorbed in the suggestions, while responding to a slight degree; but I was not hypnotized.
6. I experienced the effects of the suggestions. I was absorbed in the suggestions while responding to a moderate degree; but I was not hypnotized.
7. I experienced the effects of the suggestions. I was absorbed in the suggestions while responding to a high degree; but I was not hypnotized.

The DHRE, a modification of the DHE, measures if a client has experienced regression and/or hypnosis (Radtke and Spanos 1982).

Name _____

Description of Hypnotic Regression Experience
(Adapted from Radtke and Spanos, 1982)

Circle the item that corresponds to your experience.
1. I was not hypnotized nor regressed while responding to suggestions.
2. I experienced the effects of the suggestions. I was regressed in the suggestions, and I was hypnotized while responding to a slight degree.
3. I experienced the effects of the suggestions. I was regressed in the suggestions, and I was hypnotized while responding to a moderate degree.
4. I experienced the effects of the suggestions. I was regressed in the suggestions, and I was hypnotized while responding to a high degree.
5. I experienced the effects of the suggestions. I was regressed in the suggestions, while responding to a slight degree; but I was not hypnotized.
6. I experienced the effects of the suggestions. I was regressed in the suggestions while responding to a moderate degree; but I was not hypnotized.
7. I experienced the effects of the suggestions. I was regressed in the suggestions while responding to a high degree; but I was not hypnotized.

General Dissociation Scale (GDS)

The GDS is a DSM-IV-based measure of dissociation. Unlike the Dissociative Experiences Scale (DES), the GDS only measures dissociative pathology and not gross psychopathology.

Two hundred and five participants were given the GDS (170 female and 35 male undergraduate and graduate students between the ages of 18 and 55). Participants also completed the DES. The GDS was significantly correlated with the DES, $r = .34$, $p < .01$, and the GDS had a Cronbach's alpha of .84, p < .01. A correlation matrix was obtained for the 15 items of the GDS, and this matrix was analyzed by a principal component analysis to determine if five factors underlie this scale.

From the rotated factor matrix, Items 12, 15, 11, and 2 loaded significantly on the first factor. The respective loadings, rounded to two decimal places, were .90, -.88, .86, and -.85. Items 8, 4, 7, and 13 loaded significantly on the second factor. The respective loadings, rounded to two decimal points, were .94, -.85, .72, and -.68. Items 14, 6, 1, and 9 loaded significantly on Factor 3. And the respective loadings, rounded to two decimal places, were .92, .70, -.68, and .52.

For the fourth factor, Items 6, 3, and 5 loaded significantly on this factor. The respective loadings, rounded to two decimal points, were .57, -.86, and .84. For Factor 5, Items 7, 13, and 10 loaded significantly on this factor. And the respective loadings, rounded to two decimal places, were .47, .41, and -.93. Finally, 5 factors emerged from the principal component analysis.

Factor 1 was named dissociative fugue, and depersonalization was the name of the second factor. Factor 3 was named dissociative identity disorder, and Factor 4 was called dissociative disorder not otherwise specified. Factor 5 was called dissociative amnesia. Even though preliminary psychometric properties exist on the GDS, this instrument should be researched with a larger sample and submitted to confirmatory factor analytical analyses.

Finally, Table 1 has the items for the GDS and Table 2 has the means and standard deviations of items. Table 3 has the correlation matrix, and, finally, Table 4 has the results of the principal component analysis.

Table 1

General Dissociation Scale (GDS)

Name_____

1.   I fell the presence of two or more distinct personal identi-

ties within me, each with its own pattern of perceiving, relating, and thinking about the environment.

Not at all	Somewhat	Moderately so	Very much so
1	2	3	4

2. Two or more distinct personal identities recurrently take control of me.

Not at all	Somewhat	Moderately so	Very much so
1	2	3	4

3. My inability to recall personal information cannot be explained by ordinary forgetfulness.

Not at all	Somewhat	Moderately so	Very much so
1	2	3	4

4. My inability to recall personal information could occur even when I am not drinking, taking drugs, or taking medication.

Not at all	Somewhat	Moderately so	Very much so
1	2	3	4

5. I have persistent experiences of feeling detached from my body or mental processes.

Not at all	Somewhat	Moderately so	Very much so
1	2	3	4

6. I feel like I am in a dream world.

Not at all	Somewhat	Moderately so	Very much so
1	2	3	4

7. When I feel detached, it could or does cause impairment in my social, occupational, and other areas of functioning.

Not at all	Somewhat	Moderately so	Very much so
1	2	3	4

8. My detachment could occur even when I am not drinking, taking drugs, or taking medication.

Not at all	Somewhat	Moderately so	Very much so
1	2	3	4

9. I have trouble recalling personal information such as my name, phone number, where I live, and so forth

Not at all	Somewhat	Moderately so	Very much so
1	2	3	4

10. My ability to recall personal information could occur even when I am not drinking or on medication.
    Not at all   Somewhat   Moderately so   Very much so
        1   2   3   4

11. My ability to recall personal information could cause impairment in my social, occupational, and other areas of functioning.
    Not at all   Somewhat   Moderately so   Very much so
        1   2   3   4

12. I could have traveled away from home and could or have had difficulty remembering the past.
    Not at all   Somewhat   Moderately so   Very much so
        1   2   3   4

13. I could or have had partial or complete confusion about my identity.
    Not at all   Somewhat   Moderately so   Very much so
        1   2   3   4

14. The possibility of partial or complete confusion could occur even when I am not drinking, taking drugs, or taking medication.
    Not at all   Somewhat   Moderately so   Very much so
        1   2   3   4

15. My partial or complete confusion could cause impairment in social, occupational, and other areas of functioning.
    Not at all   Somewhat   Moderately so   Very much so
        1   2   3   4

Table 2
Means and Standard Deviations of GDS Items

	Mean	Standard Deviation
Item 1	1.07	.25
Item 2	1.51	.54
Item 3	1.18	.54
Item 4	1.18	.50
Item 5	1.08	.28
Item 6	1.17	.44
Item 7	1.22	.66
Item 8	1.13	.42
Item 9	1.07	.25
Item 10	1.11	.53
Item 11	1.15	.48
Item 12	1.14	.41
Item 13	1.17	.40
Item 14	1.15	.41
Item 15	1.21	.58

Table 3
Principle Components Analysis of GDS

1														
.332	1													
.265	.266	1												
.096	.126	.339	1											
.007	-.002	.136	.366	1										
.171	.107	.293	.431	.522	1									
.094	-.008	.520	.186	.226	.406	1								
.321	.062	.500	.373	.164	.236	.286	1							
.222	.089	.265	.387	.181	.171	.094	.610	1						
.126	.079	.156	.284	.262	.199	.048	.122	.034	1					
.369	.221	.213	.308	.355	.531	.176	.138	.116	.642	1				
.266	.267	.155	.199	.269	.369	.132	.386	.325	.122	.260	1			
.189	.179	.104	.233	.249	.276	.019	.295	.368	.051	.114	.586	1		
.253	.228	.329	.359	.413	.418	.228	.000	.001	.000	.000	.000	.000	1	
.447	.319	.297	.449	.452	.520	.099	.000	.000	.000	.000	.000	.000	.000	1

Table 4
Correlation Matrix of GDS Items

Factor Matrix:

Variable	Factor 1	Factor 2	Factor 3	Factor 4	Factor 5
G15	-.91959				
G12	.87570				
G11	.81533				
G1	-.69833				
G9	.63402				
G8	-.31501	.95115			
G4	.52880	-.87970			
G13	-.61593	-.61593			
G7	-.43972	.60267			
G10	.52012		-.75793		
G6			.75128		
G5			.71698		
G2	-.58822			-.73761	
G13	.60496			-.61943	
G3		.55981	-.34911		

Variable	Communality	*	Factor	Eigenvalue	Pct of Var	Cum Pct
G1	.77832	*	1	4.83377	32.2	32.2
G2	.99898	*	2	3.12521	20.8	53.1
G3	.97584	*	3	2.46235	16.4	69.5
G4	.99833	*	4	1.81081	12.1	81.5
G5	.84850	*	5	1.67678	11.2	92.7
G6	.99845	*				
G7	.93143					
G8	.96050					
G9	.86012					
G10	.94011					
G11	.89397					
G12	.95994					
G13	.93297					
G14	.90005					
G15	.95143					

VARIMAX rotation 1 for extraction 1 in analysis 1 - Kaiser Normalization.

VARIMAX converged in 12 iterations.

Rotated Factor Matrix:

Variable	Factor 1	Factor 2	Factor 3	Factor 4	Factor 5
G12	.89729		.26030		
G15	-.88394		-.37567		
G11	.85626		.26053		
G2	-.85034			-.32660	
G8		.93808	-.43404		
G4		-.84805	-.34931		
G7		.72456			
G13		-.68025			
G14	-.34872	.34107	.92010	.56703	
G6	.35341	-.39728	.69939		
G1			-.67939		
G9			.52154		
G3				-.86319	.28262
G5	.28552			.83344	.31737
G10					-.93028

Note: We doubled the standard error for a correlation to be significant 2(.182) = .364 for interpretation purposes.

Factor Transformation Matrix:

	Factor 1	Factor 2	Factor 3	Factor 4	Factor 5
Factor 1	.81978	-.13952	.55387	.03869	.01498
Factor 2	.16780	.93175	.00784	-.32026	.03263
Factor 3	-.12167	.21472	.17046	.63744	.70972
Factor 4	.52628	.01366	-.79655	.29705	.01060
Factor 5	.08958	-.25708	-.17212	-.63353	.70349

CHAPTER SUMMARY

This chapter described contemporary hypnosis theories and research. In addition, several instruments were provided to measure vividness of imagination, hypnotic depth, clients' misconceptions of hypnosis, absorption, dissociation, and regression. Finally, hypnosis and automaticity were discussed.

Chapter 7

PULLING IT TOGETHER: WHAT IS HYPNOSIS AND WHY IS IT RELATED TO DISSOCIATION AND ABSORPTION?

ACCORDING TO BARBER'S (1999) new 3-dimensional paradigm, the debate between the special process and nonstate theorists is no longer meaningful. He noted that most hypnosis researchers only see one of the three types of clients–fantasy-prone, amnesic-prone, or positively-set. For example, the fantasy-prone clients correspond to clients that become absorbed during hypnosis through their fantasy capacity. By the way, these are very hypnotizable clients. Similarly, the amnesic-prone clients are what Hilgard (1994) called dissociators, clients who were very hypnotizable and are spontaneously amnesic to deep levels of hypnosis. Likewise, these clients are capable of being amnesic to pain. Lastly, the positively-set clients are not as hypnotizable as the fantasy-prone or amnesic-prone, but they are able to elicit hypnosis by having positive expectancies toward hypnosis.

What, then, is hypnosis? It is the complex interplay among the three types and the dimensions of the clinician. Hypnosis occurs when a client thinks along the lines of a clinician, and the words and thoughts of the clinician become those of the client;

hence, the client is able to experience automatic ideomotor and ideosensory experiences. So, hypnosis is the complex interplay between clients' dimensions (fantasy-prone, amnesic-prone, and positively-set) and clinicians' dimensions (empathy, kinds of suggestion used, tone of suggestions, and so on).

Barber's new theory builds a bridge between special process and nonstate theories. Actually, Barber's new paradigm unifies the previous disagreements between state and nonstate theorists. One can conclude that with highly hypnotizable fantasy-prone clients, hypnotizability scores will correlate significantly with dissociation measures; therefore, clearly, dissociation and absorption are correlates of hypnotizability, but many researchers tend to measure the wrong types of clients. This is why absorption, dissociation, and hypnosis have low correlations in the literature. In addition, clients who experience dissociative disorders are highly hypnotizable amnesic-prone clients. And, finally, Barber's theory offers an explanation of why hypnosis is associated with several overlapping psychological disorders such as dissociative disorder, somatoform disorder, borderline personality disorder, posttraumatic stress disorder, and so on. Theoretically and empirically, dissociative disorders and their correlates are related to hypnosis, but due to the fact that there is a small percentage of highly hypnotizable fantasy-prone and amnesic-prone clients, clinicians may seldom see together these two types of clients. What is not explicit about Barber's new paradigm is the role of the brain in eliciting hypnosis.

Dissociated control theorists have hypothesized that the forebrain, telencephalon, which contains subcortical structures, is involved with the elicitation of hypnosis. Specifically, the frontal lobes, which are substructures of the cerebral cortex, are recently evolved parts of the brain that are associated with olfaction (smell), motor movement, and higher cognitive functions including Broca's speech area (Sapp 1997).

Logically, the midbrain, mesencephalon, has to be associated with hypnosis, because it is involved with audition (hearing), vision, sleep, arousal, and eye movements. This part of the brain could help explain how clients experience certain hypnotic phenomena such as hallucinations, regression, and so on. Furthermore, the hindbrain, metencephalon, which controls muscle coordination and receives auditory, visual, vestibular (information from the inner ear), and somatosensory information, has to be implicated with hypnosis. Clearly, there is an overlap in brain functions, and there is an overlap in theories of hypnosis; therefore, what is needed are evidence-based technically eclectic theories of the brain and hypnosis. The new brain imaging techniques such as computerized topographic scanning (CT scan), magnetic resonance imaging (MRI), and positron emission tomography (PET) will provide more specific connections between the brain and hypnosis. Finally, hypnosis is a complex phenomenon, and it will take the synthesis of several areas in order to shed more light on this elusive construct.

REFERENCES

Adrian, C. (1996). Therapist sexual feelings in hypnotherapy: Managing therapeutic boundaries in hypnotic work. *International Journal of Clinical and Experimental Hypnosis*, 44:20–32.

Arazoz, D. L. (1981). Negative self-hypnosis. *Journal of Contemporary Psychotherapy*, 12:45–52.

———(1982). *Hypnosis and sex therapy.* New York: Brunner/Mazel.

———(1985). *The new hypnosis.* New York: Brunner/Mazel.

Bandler, R., & Grinder, R. (1975). *Patterns of the hypnotic techniques of Milton H. Erickson, M.D.* Cupertino, CA: Meta Publications.

Barabasz, A., & Barabasz, M. (1996). Neurotherapy and alert hypnosis in the treatment of attention deficit/hyperactivity disorder. In I. Kirsch & J.W. Rhue (Eds.), *Casebook of Clinical Hypnosis*, pp. 271–292. Washington, DC: American Psychological Association.

Barber, J. (1998). When hypnosis causes trouble. *The International Journal of Clinical and Experimental Hypnosis*, 46:157–170.

Barber, T. X. (1969). *Hypnosis: A scientific approach.* New York: Van Nostrand Reinhold (reprinted 1995: Northvale, NJ: Jason Aronson).

———(1999). A comprehensive three-dimensional theory of hypnosis. In I. Kirsch, A. Capafons, E. Cardeña-Buelna, and S. Amigó (Eds.), *Clinical hypnosis and self-regulation*: Cognitive-Behavioral Perspectives, ed. , pp. 21–48. Washington, DC: American Psychological Association.

Barber, T. X., & Wilson, S. C. (1979). Guided imagining and hypnosis: Theoretical and empirical overlap and convergence in a new Creative Imagination Scale. In A.A. Skeikh & J.T. Shaffer (Eds.), *The potential of fantasy and imagination*, pp. 67–88. New York: Brandon House.

Bargh, J. A. (1994). The four horsemen of automaticity: Awareness, intention, efficiency, and control in social cognition. In R.S. Wyer & T.K. Srull (Eds.), *Handbook of social cognition*, (2nd ed.), pp.1–40. Hillsdale, NJ: Erlbaum.

Bargh, J. A., & Barndollar, K. (1996). Automaticity in action: The unconscious as repository of chronic goals and motives. In P.M. Gollwitzer & J.A. Bargh (Eds.) *The psychology of action: Linking cognition and motivation to behavior*, pp. 457–481. New York: Guilford.

Bargh, J. A., & Gollwitzer, P. M. (1994). Environmental control of goal-directed action: Automatic and strategic contingencies between situations and behavior. *Nebraska Symposium on Motivation*, 41:71–124.

Baron, M. (1985). Familial transmission of schizotypal and borderline personality disorders. *American Journal of Psychiatry, 142*, 927-934.

Barrett, D. (1990). Deep trance subjects: A schema of two distinct subgroups. In R.G. Kunzendorf (Ed.), *Mental imagery*, pp. 101-112. New York: Plenum Press.

⸻ (1996). Fantasizers and dissociators: Two types of high hypnotizables, two different imagery styles. In R. G. Kunzendorf, W. P. Spanos, & B. Wallace (Eds.), *Hypnosis and imagination*, , pp. 123-135. Amityville, NY: Baywood.

Bartis, S. P., & Zamansky, H. S. (1990). Cognitive strategies in hypnosis: Toward resolving the hypnotic conflict. *International Journal of Clinical and Experimental Hypnosis 38*:168-182.

Bartlett, F. C. (1932). *Remembering*. New York: Columbia University Press.

Bassman, S. (1983). *The effects of indirect hypnosis, relaxation and homework on the primary and secondary psychological symptoms of women with muscle-contraction headache*. Unpublished doctoral dissertation, University of Cincinnati, Cincinnati, OH.

Beck, A., & Weishaar, M. (1995). Current psychotherapies. In R. J. Corsini & D. Wedding, (Eds.), *Cognitive therapy*, (5th ed.), pp. 229-261. Itasca, IL: F. E. Peacock.

Benner, D. G., & Joscelyne, B. (1984). Multiple personality as a borderline disorder. *The Journal of Nervous and Mental Disease, 172*:98-104.

Bennett, H. L. (1988). Perception and memory of events during adequate general anesthesia for surgical operations. In H. M. Pettinai *Hypnosis and Memory*, pp. 193-231. New York: Guilford Press.

Bernstein, E., & Putnam, F. W. (1986). Development, reliability and validity of a dissociation scale. *Journal of Nervous and Mental Disease 174*:727-735.

Blackburn, I. M., Bishop, S., Glen, A. I. M., Whalley, L. J., & Christie, J. E. (1981). The efficacy of cognitive therapy in depression: A treatment trial using cognitive therapy and pharmacotherapy, each alone and in combination. *British Journal of Psychiatry, 139*:181-189.

Bothwell, R. K., Deffenbacher, K. A., & Brigham, J. C. (1987). Correlation of eyewitness accuracy and confidence: Optimality hypothesis revisited. *Journal of Applied Psychology, 72*:691-695.

Bowers, K. S. (1993). The Waterloo-Stanford Group C (WSGC) scale of hypnotic susceptibility: Normative and comparative data. *International Journal of Clinical and Experimental Hypnosis, 41*:35-46.

⸻ (1998). Waterloo-Stanford Group Scale of Hypnotic

Susceptibility, Form C; Manual and response booklet. *International Journal of Clinical and Experimental Hypnosis 46*:250-268.

Braun, B. G. (1988). The BASK model of dissociation. *Dissociation, 1*:4-23.

Braun, B. G., and Sachs, R. G. (1985). The development of multiple personality disorder: Predisposing precipitating and perpetuating factors. In R. P. Kluft (Ed.), *Childhood antecedents of multiple personality*, pp. 38-64. Washington, DC: American Psychiatric Press.

Brewster, W. F., & Treyens, J. C. (1981). Role of schemata in memory for places. *Cognitive Psychology, 13*:207-230.

Cardeña, E. (1994). The domain of dissociation. In S. J. Lynn and J. W. Rhue (Eds.), *Dissociation: clinical and theoretical perspectives*, pp. 15-31. New York Guilford Press.

Chaves, J. F., & Dworkin, S. F. (1997). Hypnotic control of pain: Historical perspectives and future prospects. *International Journal of Clinical and Experimental Hypnosis, 14*:356-376.

Clary, W. F., Burstein, K. J., & Carpenter, J. S. (1984). Multiple personality and borderline personality disorder. *Psychiatric Clinics of North America 7*:89-99.

Coe, W. C., & Sarbin, T. R. (1991). Role theory: Hypnosis from a dramaturgical and narrational perspective. In S. J. Lynn and J. W. Rhue, (Eds.). *Theories of hypnosis: current models and perspectives*, pp. 303-323. New York: Guilford Press.

Coe, W., & Scharcoff, J. (1985). An empirical evaluation of the neurolinguistic programming model. *International Journal of Clinical and Experimental Hypnosis, 23*:310-319.

Connery, D. S. (1982). *The inner source: Exploring hypnosis with Dr. Herbert Spiegel.* New York: Holt, Rinehart and Winston.

Coryell, W. (1983). Multiple personality and primary affective disorder. *Journal of Nervous and Mental Disease, 171*:388-390.

Council, J. R. (1999). Measures of hypnotic responding. In I. Kirsch, A. Capafons, E. Cardeña- Buelna, & S. Amigó (Eds.), *Clinical hypnosis and self-regulation: Cognitive-behavioral perspectives*, pp. 119-140. Washington, DC: American Psychological Association.

Diagnostic and Statistical Manual of Mental Disorders (1994) (4th ed.). Washington, DC: American Psychiatric Association.

Dinges, D. F., Whitehouse, W. G., Orne, E. C., Bloom, P. R., Carlin, M. M., Bauer, N. K., & Gillen, K. A. (1997). Self-hypnosis training as an adjunctive treatment in the management of pain associated with sickle cell disease. *International Journal of Clinical and Experimental Hypnosis, 14*:417-432.

Dixon, M., & Laurence, J. R. (1992). Hypnotic susceptibility and verbal automaticity: Automatic and strategic processing differences in the Stroop color-naming task. *Journal of Abnormal Psychology, 101*:344–347.

Dixon, M., Brunet, A., & Laurence, J. R. (1990). Hypnotizability and automaticity: Toward a parallel distributed processing model of hypnotic responding. *Journal of Abnormal Psychology, 99*:336–343.

Dobson, K. S. (1989). A meta-analysis of efficacy of cognitive therapy for depression. *Journal of Consulting and Clinical Psychology, 57*:414–419.

Dowd, E. T., & Hingst, A. G. (1983). Matching therapists' predicates: An in vivo test of effectiveness. *Perceptual Motor Skills, 57*:207–210.

Dowd, E. T., & Petty, J. (1982). Effect of counselor predicate matching on perceived social influence and client satisfaction. *Journal of Counseling Psychology, 29*:206-209.

Edgette, J. H., & Edgette, J. S. (1995). *The handbook of hypnotic phenomena in psychotherapy.* New York: Brunner/Mazel.

Edmonston, W. E. (1986). *The induction of hypnosis.* New York: John Wiley and Sons.

Edmonston, W. F., Jr. (1981). *Hypnosis and relaxation: Modern verification of an old equation.* New York: Wiley.

——— (1991). Anesis. In S. J. Lynn & J. W. Rhue (Eds.), *Theories of hypnosis: Current models and perspectives,* pp. 197–240. New York: Guilford.

Ellenberger, H. F. (1970). *The discovery of the unconscious: The history and evolution of dynamic psychiatry.* New York: Basic Books.

Ellis, A. (1993). Fundamentals of rational-emotive therapy. In W. Dryden & L. K. Hills (Eds.), *Innovations in rational-emotive therapy,* pp. 1–32. Newbury Park, CA: SAGE.

Erdelyi, M. H. (1995). Repression, reconstruction, and defense: History and integration of the psychoanalytic and experimental frameworks. In J. L. Singer *Repression and dissociation: Implications for personality theory, psychopathology, and health,* pp. 1–32. Chicago: University Press of Chicago.

Erickson, M. H., & Rossi, E. (1979). *Hypnotherapy: An exploratory casebook.* New York: Irvington.

——— (Eds.) (1980). *The collected papers of Milton H. Erickson on hypnosis: Vol. I. The nature of hypnosis and suggestion.* New York: Irvington.

——— (1981). *Experiencing hypnosis.* New York: Irvington.

——— (1989). *The February Man.* New York: Irvington.

Erickson, M. H., Rossi, S. I., & Rossi, E. L. (1976). *Hypnotic realities.* New York: Irvington.

Evers-Szostak, M., & Sanders, S. (1992). The Children's Perceptual

Alteration Scale (PAS): A measure of children's dissociation. *Dissociation*, 5:91–97.

Faith, M., & Ray, W. (1994). Hypnotizability and dissociation in a college-age population: Orthogonal individual differences. *Personality and Individual Differences*, 17:211–216.

Farthing, G. H., Venturino, M., Brown, S. W., & Lazar, J. D. (1997). Internal and external distraction in the control of cold-pressor pain as a function of hypnotizability. *International Journal of Clinical and Experimental Hypnosis*, 14:433–446.

Fink, D. (1991). The comorbidity of multiple personality disorder and DSM-III-R axis II disorders. *Psychiatric Clinics of North American* 14:547–566.

Fourie, D. P. (1991). The ecosystem approach to hypnosis. In S. J. Lynn and J. W. Rhue (Eds.), *Theories of hypnosis*, pp. 467–484. New York: Guilford Press.

Fromm, E, & Nash, M. (1997). *Psychoanalysis and hypnosis.* Madison, CT: International Universities Press.

Fyer, M. R. (1988). Comorbidity of borderline personality disorder. *Archives of General Psychiatry*, 45:348–352.

Gibbons, D. E. (1979). *Applied hypnosis and hyperemperia.* New York: Plenum.

Gill, M. M., & Brenman, M. (1959). *Hypnosis and related states: Psychoanalytic studies in regression.* Madison, CT: International Universities Press.

Glass, L. B., & Barber, T. X. (1961). A note on hypnotic behavior, the definition of the situation, and the placebo effect. *Journal of Nervous and Mental Diseases* 132:539–541.

Granvold, D. K. (Ed.) (1994). *Cognitive and behavioral treatment: methods and applications.* Pacific Grove, CA: Brooks/Cole.

Gravitz, M. A. (1991). Early theories of hypnosis: A clinical perspective. In S. J. Lynn and J. W. Rhue (Eds.), Theories of hypnosis: Current models and perspectives, pp. 19–42.

Green, J. P. (1999). Hypnosis and the treatment of smoking cessation and weight loss. In I. Kirsch, A. Capanafons, E. Cardeña-buelna, & S. Amigó (Eds.), *Clinical Hypnosis and Self-Regulation: Cognitive-Behavioral Perspectives*, pp. 249–276. Washington, DC: American Psychological Association.

Grinder, J., DeLozier, J., & Bandler, R. (1977). *Patterns of the hypnotic technique of Milton H. Erickson, M.D., vol. 2.* Cupertino, CA: Meta Publications.

Gruenewald, D., Fromm, E., & Oberlander, M. I. (1979). Hypnosis and adaptive regression. An ego-psychological inquiry. In E. Fromm and R. E. Shore (Eds.), *Hypnosis: research developments and new perspectives*, pp. 619-636. Chicago: Aldine..

Gumm, W. B., Walker, M. K., & Day, H. D. (1982). Neurolinguistic programming: Method or myth? *Journal of Counseling Psychology*, 29:327–330.

Gunderson, J. G. (1984). *Borderline personality disorder.* Washington, DC: American Psychiatric Press.

Hadfield, J. A. (1967). *Introduction to psychotherapy: Its history and Modern schools.* London: George Allen and Unwin.

Haley, J. (Ed.) (1967). *Advanced techniques of hypnosis and therapy: Selected papers of Milton H. Erickson, M.D.* New York: Grune and Stratton.

——— (1973). *Uncommon therapy: The psychiatric techniques of Milton H. Erickson, M.D.* New York: Norton.

Hammond, C. D. (1992). Hypnotic Induction and Suggestion: An Introductory Manual. Des Plaines, IL: American Society of Clinical Hypnosis.

Hargadon, R., Bowers, K. S., & Woody, E. Z. (1995). Does counterpain imagery mediate hypnotic analgesia? *Journal of Abnormal Psychology* 104:508–516.

Hartland, J. (1966). *Medical and dental hypnosis.* London: Bailliere.

Henry, D. (1984). *The neurolinguistic programming construct of the primary representational system: A multitrait multimethod validational study.* Unpublished master's thesis, University of Connecticut, Storrs, CT.

Hergenhahn, B. R. (1997). *An introduction to the history of psychology.* Pacific Grove, CA: Brooks/Cole.

Hilgard, E. R. (1965). *Hypnotic susceptibility.* New York: Harcourt Brace Jovanovich.

———(1991). A neodissociation interpretation of hypnosis. In S. J. Lynn and J. W. Rhue (Eds.), *Theories of Hypnosis: Current Models and Perspectives*, pp. 32–51. New York: Guilford Press.

———(1994). Neodissociation theory. In S. J. Lynn and J. W. Rhue (Eds.), *Dissociation: clinical and theoretical perspectives* (pp. 83-104). New York: Guilford.

Hilgard, E. R., & Hilgard, J. R. (1975). *Hypnosis in relief of pain.* Los Altos, CA: Kaufmann.

———(1994). *Hypnosis in the relief of pain,* (Rev. ed.) New York: Brunner/Mazel.

Hilgard, J. R. (1974). Imaginative involvement: Some characteristics of highly hypnotizable and nonhypnotizable. *International Journal of Clinical and Experimental Hypnosis,* 22:138-156.

Horevitz, R. P. (1996). The treatment of a case of dissociative identity disorder. In S. J. Lynne, I. Kirsch, and J. W. Rhue (Eds.), *Casebook of clinical hypnosis,* pp. 193-222. Washington, DC: American Psychology Association.

Horevitz, R. P., & Braun, B. G. (1984). Are multiple personalities borderline? *Psychiatric Clinics of North America,* 7:69-72.

Hornstein, N. L. (1993). Recognition and differential diagnosis of dissociative disorders in children and adolescents. *Dissociation,* 2:136-144.

Katz, N. (1979). Comparative efficacy of behavioral training, training plus relaxation, and a sleep/trance induction in increasing hypnotic susceptibility. *Journal of Consulting and Clinical Psychology,* 47:119-127.

Kirsch, I. (1990). *Changing expectations: A key to effective psychotherapy.* Pacific Grove, CA: Brooks/Cole.

——— (1991). The social learning theory of hypnosis. In S. J. Lynn & J. W. Rhue, (Eds.), *Theories of Hypnosis: Current Models and Perspectives,* pp. 439-465. New York: Guilford Press.

——— (1993). Cognitive-behavioral hypnotherapy. In J. W. Rhue, S. J. Lynn, and I. Kirsch (Eds.), *Handbook of clinical hypnosis,* pp. 439-466. Washington, DC: American Psychological Association.

——— (1996). Dissociation: Dissociated and reassociated. Review of the book *Dissociation: Clinical and Theoretical Perspectives. Contemporary Psychology* 41:260-262

——— (1997). Response expectancy and application: A decennial review. *Applied and Preventive Psychology,* 6:69-79.

Kirsch, I, Burgess, C. A., & Braffman, W. (1999). Attentional resources in hypnotic responding. *International Journal of Clinical and Experimental Hypnosis,* 47:175-191.

Kirsch, I., and Lynn, S. J. (1995). The altered state of hypnosis: Changes in the theoretical landscape. *American Psychology,* 50:846-858.

——— (1997). Hypnotic involuntariness and the automaticity of everyday life. *American Journal of Clinical Hypnosis,* 40:329-349.

——— (1998a). Dissociation theories of hypnosis. *Psychological Bulletin,* 123:100-115.

——— (1998b). Social-cognitive alternatives to dissociation theories of hypnotic involuntariness. *Review of General Psychology,* 2:66-80.

——— (1999). Automaticity in clinical psychology. *American Psychologists,* 54:504-515.

Kirsch, I., Mobayed, C. P., Council, J. R., & Kenny, D. A. (1992). Expert judgments of hypnosis from subjective state reports. *Journal of Abnormal Psychology, 101*:657–662.

Kirsch, I., Montgomery, G., and Sapirstein, G. (1995). Hypnosis as an adjunct to cognitive behavioral psychotherapy: A meta-analysis. *Journal of Consulting and Clinical Psychology, 63*:214–220.

Kluft, R. P. (1982). Varieties of hypnotic interventions in the treatment of multiple personality. *American Journal of Clinical Hypnosis, 24*:230–240.

———(1984). The treatment of multiple personality disorder. *Psychiatric Clinics of North America, 7*:9–30.

———(1990). The diagnosis and treatment of multiple personality disorder. *Directions in Clinical Psychology, 3*:3–55.

———(1991). Clinical presentations of multiple personality disorder. *Psychiatric Clinics of North America, 14*:605–630.

Knapp, S., & Vande Creek, L. (1996). Risk management for psychologists: Treating patients who recover lost memories of child abuse. *Professional Psychology: Research and Practice 27*:452–459.

Kreisman, J. J., & Straus, H. (1989). *I hate you–Don't leave me: Understanding the borderline personality*. New York: Avon Books.

Laurence, J. R., & Perry, C. (1983). Hypnotically created pseudo memories among highly hypnotizable subjects. *Science, 222*:523–524.

LeCron, L. M. (1954). A hypnotic technique for uncovering unconscious material. *Journal of Clinical and Experimental Hypnosis, 2*:76–79.

Levitt, E. E. (1993). Hypnosis in the treatment of obesity. In J. W. Rhue, S. J. Lynn, and I. Kirsch (Eds.), *Handbook of clinical hypnosis*, pp. 533–554. Washington DC: American Psychological Association.

Libet, B. (1985). Unconscious cerebral initiative and the role of conscious will in voluntary action. *Behavioral and Brain Sciences, 8*:529–566.

Loftus, E. R. (1979). *Eyewitness testimony*. Cambridge, MA: Harvard University Press.

———(1993). The reality of repressed memories. *American Psychologist, 48*:518–537.

London, P. (1963). *Children's hypnotic susceptibility scale*. Palo Alto, CA: Consulting Psychological Press.

Loranger, A., Oldham, J., & Tulis, E. (1982). Familial transmission of DSM-III borderline personality disorder. *Archives of General Psychiatry, 39*:795–799.

Lynn, S. J. (1992). A non-state of hypnotic involuntariness. *Contemporary Hypnosis, 9*:21–27.

Lynn, S. J., Neufeld, V., & Maré, C. (1993). Direct versus indirect suggestions: A conceptual and methodological review. *International Journal of Clinical and Experimental Hypnosis, 41*:124–152.

Lynn, S. J., & Rhue, J. W. (Eds.) (1991). *Theories of hypnosis: Current models and perspectives.* New York: Guilford Press.

——— (1994). *Dissociation: Clinical and theoretical perspectives.* New York: Guilford Press.

Mandler, J. N. (1984). *Stories, scripts, and scenes: Aspects of schema theory.* Hillsdale, NJ: Erlbaum.

Masters, R. (1978). *How your mind can keep you well.* Los Angeles: Foundation of Human Understanding.

McConkey, K. M. (1984). The impact of indirect suggestion. *International Journal of Clinical and Experimental Hypnosis, 32*:307–314.

——— (1986). Opinions about hypnosis and self-hypnosis before and after hypnotic testing. *International Journal of Clinical and Experimental Hypnosis, 34*:311–319.

Morgan, A. H., & Hilgard, E. R. (1973). Age differences in susceptibility to hypnosis. *International Journal of Clinical and Experimental Hypnosis, 21*:781–785.

Nace, E. P., Saxon, J., & Shore, N. (1983). A comparison of borderline and non-borderline alcoholic patients. *Archives of General Psychiatry, 40*:54–56.

Nash, M. R. (1987). What, if anything, is regressed about hypnotic age regression? A review of the empirical literature. *Psychological Bulletin, 102*:42–52.

——— (1991). Hypnosis as a special case of psychological regression. In S. J. Lynn & J. W. Rhue (Eds.), *Theories of Hypnosis: Current Models and Perspectives*, pp. 171–196). New York: Guilford Press.

Nash, M. R., Hulsey, T. L., Sexton, M. C., Harralson, T. L., & Lambert, W. (1993). Long-term sequelae of childhood sex abuse: Perceived family environment, psychopathology, and dissociation. *Journal of Consulting and Clinical Psychology, 61*:276–283.

Nash, M. R., Lynn, S. L., & Givens, D. L. (1984). Adult hypnotic susceptibility, childhood punishment, and child abuse: A brief communication. *International Journal of Clinical and Experimental Hypnosis, 32*:6–11.

Neisser, U., & Harsch, N. (1992). Phantom flashbulbs: False recollections of hearing the news about Challenger. In E. Winograd and U. Neisser (Eds.), *affect and accuracy in recall: Studies of "flashbulb" memories*, pp. 9–31. New York: Cambridge University Press.

Neisser, U. (1976). *Cognition and reality*. San Francisco: Freeman.
Norman, D. A., & Shallice, T. (1986). Attention to action: Willed and automatic control of behavior. In R. J. Davidson, G. E. Schwartz *Consciousness and self-regulation*, vol. 4. pp. 1–18. New York: Plenum Press.
Orne, M. T. (1979). On the simulating subject as a quasi-control group in hypnosis research: What, why and how. In E. Fromm and R. E. Shor (Eds.), *Hypnosis: Developments in research and new perspectives*, 2nd ed., pp. 519–565. Chicago: Aldine.
Orne, M. T., & Dinges, D. F. (1984). Hypnosis. In P. D. Wall and R. Melzack (Eds.), *Textbook of pain*, pp. 806–817. New York: Churchill Livingstone.
Page, R. A., Hanley, G. W., & Green, J. P. (1997). Response expectancies and beliefs about hypnosis: Another look. *Contemporary Hypnosis*, 14:173–181.
Pashler, H. E. (1998). *The psychology of attention*. Cambridge, MA: The MIT Press.
Patterson, D. R., Adcock, R. J., & Bombardier, C H. (1997). Factors predicting hypnotic analgesia in clinical burn pain. *International Journal of Clinical and Experimental Hypnosis*, 14:377–395.
Pekala, R. J., Kumar, V. K., & Marcano, G. (1995). Hypnotic types: A partial replication concerning phenomenal experience. *Contemporary Hypnosis*, 12:194–200.
Perry, C. (1978). The Abbé Faria: A neglected figure in the history of hypnosis. In F. H. Frankel and H. S. Zamansky (Eds.), *Hypnosis at its bicentennial*, pp. 37–46. New York: Plenum Press.
Perry, C., Gelfand, R., & Marcovitch, P. (1979). The relevance of hypnotic susceptibility in the clinical context. *Journal of Abnormal Psychology*, 88:592–603.
Perry, C., Nadon, R., & Button, J. (1992). The measurement of hypnotic ability. In E. Fromm and M. R. Nash (Eds.), *Contemporary hypnosis research*, pp. 459–498. New York: Guilford Press.
Piaget, J. (1926). *The language and thought of the child*. New York: Harcourt, Brace.
Piccione, C., Hilgard, E. R., & Zimbardo, P. G. (1989). On the degree of stability of measured hypnotizability over a 25-year period. *Journal of Personality and Social Psychology*, 56:289–295.
Putnam, F. W. (1991). Childhood MPD proposal. Unpublished data in R. P. Kluft (1984), Multiple personality in childhood. *Psychiatric Clinics of North America*, 7:121–134.

———(1994). Dissociative disorders in children and adolescents. In *Dissociation: Clinical and Theoretical Perspectives*, ed. S. J. Lynn and J. W. Rhue, pp. 175-189. New York: Guilford.

Putnam, F. W., Guroff, J. J., Silberman, E. K., Barban, L., and Post, R. M. (1986). The clinical phenomenology of multiple personality disorder: A review of 100 recent cases. *Journal of Clinical Psychiatry* 47:285-293.

Putnam, F. W., Helmers, K., and Trickett, P. D. (1993). Development, reliability and validity of a child dissociation scale. *Child Abuse and Neglect* 17:731-741.

Radtke, H. L., & Spanos, N. P. (1982). The effect of rating scale descriptors on hypnotic depth reports. *Journal of Psychology, 111*:235-245.

Reagor, P. A., Kasten, J. D., & Morelli, N. (1992). A checklist for screening dissociative disorders in children and adolescents. *Dissociation ,5*:4-19.

Richardson, L. F. (1998). Psychogenic dissociation in childhood: The role of the counseling psychologist. *The Counseling Psychologist, 26*:69-100.

Roche, S., & McConkey, K. M. (1990). Absorption: Nature, assessment, & correlates. *Journal of Personality and Social Psychology, 59*:91-101.

Ross, C. A. (1989). *Multiple personality disorder: Diagnosis, clinical features, and treatment.* New York: Wiley.

Sanders, B. (1992). The imaginary companion experience in multiple personality disorder. *Dissociation, 5*:159-162.

Sapp, M. (1995). Hypnosis: Applications for clients with physical disabilities who are seeking supported employment. *The Australian Journal of Clinical Hypnotherapy and Hypnosis, 16*:1-8.

———(1996). Potential negative sequelae of hypnosis. *The Australian Journal of Clinical Hypnotherapy and Hypnosis, 17*:73-77.

———(1997a). Order effects for two measures of hypnotizability. *Perceptual and Motor Skills, 83*:1-42.

———(1997b). *Counseling and psychotherapy: Theories, associated research, and issues.* Lanham, MD: University Press of America.

———(1997c). *General dissociation scale.* Unpublished manuscript.

———(1997d). Hypnotizability Scales: What are they and are they useful? *The Australian Journal of Clinical Hypnotherapy and Hypnosis, 18*: 25-31.

———(1999). *Test anxiety: Applied research, assessment, and treatment interventions.* Lanham, MD: University Press of America.

Sapp, M., and Evanow, M. (1998). Hypnotizability: Absorption and dissociation. The Australian *Journal of Clinical Hypnotherapy and Hypnosis,* 19:1–8.

Sapp, M., Evanow, M., & Arndt, M. (1997). *Hypnotizability: Absorption and dissociation.* Paper presented at the Annual Convention of the American Psychological Association, Chicago.

Sapp, M., Farrell, W., Johnson, J., Sartin-Kirby, R., & Pumphrey, K. (1997). Hypnosis: Applications for rehabilitation. *Journal of Applied Rehabilitation Counseling,* 28:31–37.

Sapp, M., Ioannidis, G., & Farrell, W. (1995). Posttraumatic stress disorder, imaginative involvement, hypnotic susceptibility, anxiety, and depression in college students. *The Australian Journal of Clinical Hypnotherapy and Hypnosis,* 16:75–88.

Sarbin, T. R. (1999). Believed-in imaginings: A narrative approach. In J. de Rivera and T. R. Sarb (Eds.), in*Believed-in imaginings: The narrative construction reality,* pp. 15–30. Washington, DC: American Psychological Association.

Sarbin, T. R., & Coe, W. E. (1972). *Hypnosis: A social psychological analysis of influence communication.* New York: Holt, Rinehart and Winston.

Sarbin, T. R., & Slagle, R. W. (1979). Hypnosis and psychophysiological outcomes. In E. Fromm and R. E. Shore (Eds.), *Hypnosis: Developments in research and new perspectives,* rev. ed., pp. 81–103. Chicago: Aldine.

Schilder, P. F. (1956). *The Nature of hypnosis* (G. Corvin, Trans.). New York: International Press.

Sheehan, P. W., & McConkey, K. M. (1982). *Hypnosis and experience: The exploration of phenomena and process.* Hillsdale, NJ: Erlbaum.

Shor, R. E., & Orne, E. C. (1962). *Harvard group scale of hypnotic susceptibility.* Palo Alto, CA: Consulting Psychologists Press.

Shor, R. E. (1959). Hypnosis and concept of the generalized reality orientation. *American Journal of Psychotherapy,* 13:582–602.

Singer, J. L. (1990). *Repression and dissociation: Implications for personality pheory, psychopathology, and health.* Chicago: The University of Chicago Press.

Spanos, N. P. (1986). Hypnotic behavior: A social psychological interpretation of amnesia, analgesia and "trance logic." *Behavioral and Brain Sciences,* 9:489–497.

———(1991). A sociocognitive approach to hypnosis. In S. J. Lynn and J. W. Rhue (Eds.), *Theories of hypnosis: Current models and perspectives,* pp. 324–361. New York: Guilford Press.

———(1996). *Multiple identities and false memories: A sociocognitive perspective.* Washington, DC: American Psychological Association.

Spanos, N. P., Radtke, H. L., Hodgins, D. C., Stam, H. J., & Bertrand, L.

D. (1983). The Carleton University Responsiveness to Suggestion Scale: Normative data and psychometric properties. *Psychological Reports*, *53*:523–535.

Spiegel, D. (1998). Hypnosis and implicit memory: Automatic processing of explicit comment. *American Journal of Clinical Hypnosis*, *40*:231–240.

Spiegel, H., & Spiegel, D. (1978). *Trance and treatment: Clinical uses of hypnosis*. New York: Basic Books.

Steinberg, M. (1996). The psychological assessment of dissociation. In L. K. Michelson and W. Ray (Eds.), *Handbook of dissociation: Theoretical, empirical, and clinical perspectives*, pp. 251–268. New York: Plenum Press.

Stern, J. A., Brown, M., Ulett, G. A., & Sletten, I. (1977). A comparison of hypnosis, acupuncture, morphine, Valium, aspirin, and placebo in the management of experimentally induced pain. *Annals of the New York Academy of Science*, *296*:175–193.

Tan, S., & Leucht, C. A. (1997). Cognitive-behavioral therapy for clinical pain control: A 15 year update and its relationship to hypnosis. *International Journal of Clinical and Experimental Hypnosis*, *14*:396–416.

Tellegen, A., & Atkinson, G. (1974). Openness to absorbing and self-altering experiences ("absorption"), a trait related to hypnotic susceptibility. *Journal of Abnormal Psychology*, *83*:268–277.

Tyson, G. M. (1992). Childhood MPD/dissociative identity disorder: Applying and extending current diagnostic checklists. *Dissociation*, *5*:20–27.

Van Gorp, W. G., Myer, R. G., & Dunbar, K. D. (1985). The efficacy of direct versus indirect hypnotic induction techniques or reduction of experimental pain. *International Journal of Clinical and Experimental Hypnosis*, *4*:319–328.

Van Den Hout, M., & Merckelbach, H. (1991). Classical conditioning: Still going strong. *Behavioral Psychotherapy*, *19*:59–79.

Vickery, A. R., Kirsch, I., Council, J. R., & Sirkin, M. I. (1985). Cognitive skill and traditional trance hypnotic inductions: A within-subjects comparison. *Journal of Consulting and Clinical Psychology*, *53*:131–133.

Wagstaff, G. F. (1991). Compliance, belief, and semantic in hypnosis: A nonstate sociocognitive perspective. In S. J. Lynn and J. W. Rhue (Eds.), *Theories of hypnosis: Current models and perspectives*, pp. 362–396. New York: Guilford Press.

Waller, N. G., Putnam, F. W., & Carlson, E. B. (1996). Types of dissociation and dissociative types: A taxometric analysis of dissociative experiences. *Psychological Methods, 1*:300–321.

Watson, R. I. (1978). *The great psychologists* (2nd ed.). Philadelphia: Lippincott.

Wegner, D. (1994). Ironic processes of mental control. *Psychological Review, 101*:34–52.

Wegner, D., and Wheatley, T. (1999). Apparent mental causation: Sources of the experience of will. *American Psychologists ,54*:480–492.

Weitzenhoffer, A. M. (1978). What did he (Bernhein) say? In F. H. Frankel and H. S. Zamansky (Eds., *Hypnosis at its bicentennial*, pp. 47–58. New York: Plenum Press.

Weitzenhoffer, A. M., & Hilgard, E. R. (1959). *Stanford Hypnotic Susceptibility Scale, Form A & B*. Palo Alto, CA: Consulting Psychologists Press.

——— (1967). *Revised Stanford Profile Scales of Hypnotic Susceptibility, Forms I and II*. Palo Alto, CA: Consulting Psychologists press.

Wells, G. L. (1993). What do we know about eye witness identification? *American Psychologist, 48*:553–571.

Wells, G. L., & Murray, D. M. (1984). Eyewitness confidence. In, ed. G. L. Wells and E. F. Loftus (Eds.), *Eyewitness Testimony: Psychological Perspectives*, pp. 155–170. New York: Cambridge University Press.

Whalen, J. E., & Nash, M. R. (1996). Hypnosis and dissociation. In , ed. L. K. Michelson and W. Ray (Eds.), *Handbook of dissociation: Theoretical, empirical, and clinical perspectives*, pp. 191-206. New York: Plenum Press.

Wickless, C., & Kirsch, I. (1989). The effects of verbal and experiential expectancy manipulations on hypnotic susceptibility. *Journal of Personality and Social Psychology, 57*:762–768.

Wilber, C. B. (1986). Psychoanalysis and multiple personality disorder. In B. G. Braun (Ed.), *The treatment of multiple personality disorder*, pp. 1–50. Washington, DC: American Psychiatric Press.

Wilson, S. C., & Barber, T. X. (1981). Vivid fantasy and hallucinatory abilities in life histories of excellent hypnotic subjects ("somnambules"): Preliminary report with female subjects. In E. Klinger (Ed.), *Imagery: Concepts, results, and applications*, pp. 133–149. New York: Plenum Press.

Wilson, S. C., & Barber, T. X. (1983). The fantasy-prone personality: Implications for understanding imagery, hypnosis, and parapsychological phenomena. In A. A. Sheikh (Ed.), *Imagery: Current theory, research, and application*, pp. 340–387. New York: Wiley.

Woody, E., & Farvolden, P. (1998). Dissociation in hypnosis and frontal executive function. *American Journal of Clinical Hypnosis, 40*:206–216.

Woody, E. Z., & Bowers, K. S. (1994). A frontal assault on dissociated control. In S. J. Lynn and J. W. Rhue (Eds.), *Dissociation: Clinical, theoretical and research perspectives*, pp. 52–79. New York: Guilford Press.

Yant, M. (1992). *Presumed guilty: When innocent people are wrongly convicted.* Buffalo, NY: Prometheus.

Yapko, M. D. (1996). A brief therapy approach to the use of hypnosis in treating depression. In S. L. Lynn, I. Kirsch, and J. W. Rhue (Eds.), *Casebook of clinical hypnosis*, pp. 75–98. Washington, DC: American Psychological Association.

Zeig, J. K., & Rennick, P. T. (1991). Ericksonian hypnotherapy: A communications approach to hypnosis. In S. J. Lynn and J. W. Rhue (Eds.), *Theories of hypnosis: Current models and perspectives*, pp. 275–302. New York: Guilford.

AUTHOR INDEX

A

Adcock, R. J., 4
Adian, C., 98, 99
Araoz, D. L., 76
Arndt, M., 21
Atkinson, G., 34

B

Bandler, R., 28, 29
Barabasz, A., 32, 67, 92
Barabasz, M., 32, 67, 92
Barban, L., 49
Barber, J., 33
Barber, T. X., 10, 87, 102, 103, 106, 112, 134–36
Bargh, J. A., 115, 117
Barlett, F. C., 117
Barndollar, K., 115, 117
Baron, M., 42
Barrett, D., 104
Bartis, S. P., 120
Bassman, S., 72
Beck, A., 92
Benner, D. G., 48
Bennett, H. L., 24
Bernstein, E., 51
Bertrand, L. D., 112
Blackburn, I. M., 92
Bombardier, C. H., 4
Bothwell, R. K., 114
Bowers, K. S., 26, 31, 103, 110, 121

Braffman, W., 32
Braun, B. G., 48, 53
Brenman, M., 35, 78
Brewster, W. F., 114
Brown, M., 4
Brown, S. W., 4
Brunet, A., 117
Burgess, C., 32
Burstein, K. J., 48

C

Carlson, E. B., 22
Carpenter, J. S., 48
Chaves, J. F., 4
Christie, J. E., 92
Clary, W. F., 48
Coe, W. E., 10, 29, 33, 106
Connery, D. C., 106
Coryell, W., 48
Council, J. R., 33, 34, 108, 111, 112

D

Day, H. D., 29
Deffenbacher, K. A., 114
De Lozier, J., 28
Dinges, D. F., 4
Dixon, M., 117
Dobson, K. S., 92
Dowd, E. T., 29
Dunbar, K. D., 29
Dworkin, S. F., 4

E

Edmonston, W. E., 12, 26, 36, 78
Edgette, J. H., 27
Edgette, J. S., 27
Ellis, A., 76
Erdelyi, M. H., 22
Erickson, M. H., 24, 26, 27, 29, 70
Evanow, M., 21, 50, 109
Evers-Szostak, M., 57

F

Faith, M., 50
Farrell, W., 17, 33, 96
Farthing, G. H., 4
Farvolden, P., 115, 116, 120
Fourie, D. P., 118
Fromm, E., 35, 45, 78
Fyer, M. R., 42

G

Gelfand, R., 4
Gibbons, D. E., 92
Gill, M. M., 35, 78
Givens, D. L., 50
Glass, L. B., 33
Glen, A. I. M., 92
Gollwitzer, P. M., 117
Granvold, D. K., 117
Gravitz, M. A., 12
Green, J. P., 95, 117, 123
Grinder, R., 28, 29
Gruenewald, D., 35
Gumm, W. B., 29
Gunderson, J. G., 42
Guroff, J. J., 49

H

Hadfield, J. A., 16, 17

Haley, J., 28
Hanley, G. W., 117
Hammond, C. D., 25
Hargadon, R., 121
Harralson, T. L., 51
Harsch, N., 114
Hartland, J., 75
Henry, D., 29
Hergenhahn, B. R., 6
Hilgard, E. R., 4, 30, 87, 102, 103, 111, 121
Hilgard, J. R., 4, 20, 26, 103, 109, 111, 115, 116, 120, 134
Hingst, A. G., 29
Hodgins, D. C., 112
Horevitz, R. P., 48
Horney, K., 14
Horstein, N. L., 56
Hulsey, T. L., 51

I

Ioannidis, G., 17

J

Johnson, J., 17, 33, 96
Joscelyne, B., 48

K

Kasten, J. D., 55
Katz, N., 33
Kenny, D. A., 34
Kirsch, I., 19, 20, 27, 30, 33, 34, 106, 108, 115, 117–21
Kirsch, J. T., 32
Kluft, R. P., 46, 48, 49, 53, 54, 56
Knapp, S., 56
Kreisman, J. J., 42
Kumar, V. K., 106

Author Index

L

Lambert, W., 51
Laurence, J. R., 117
Lazar, J. D., 4
LeCron, L. M., 24
Leucht, C. A., 4
Levitt, E. E., 95
Libet, B., 119
Loftus, E. R., 114
London, P., 111
Loranger, A., 42
Lynn, S. J., 27, 30, 31, 33, 50, 106, 115, 117, 119–21

M

Mandler, J. N., 114
Marcano, G., 106
Marcovitch, P., 4
Maré, C., 27
Masters, R., 72, 74
McConkey, K. M., 20, 21, 29, 33, 106, 111
Merkelbach, H., 117
Mobayed, C. P., 34
Morgan, A. H., 4
Morelli, N., 55
Murray, D. N., 114
Myer, R. G., 29

N

Nash, M. R., 25, 26, 34, 35, 45, 50, 51, 78
Neisser, U., 114
Neufeld, V., 27
Norman, D. A., 117, 120

O

Oberlander, M. I., 35

Oldham, J., 42
Orne, E. C., 4, 34

P

Page, R. A., 117, 123
Pashler, H. E., 121
Patterson, D. R., 4
Pekala, R. J., 106
Perry, C., 4, 111
Petty, J., 29
Piaget, J., 118
Piccione, C., 102, 109, 121
Post, R. M., 49
Pumphrey, K., 17, 33, 96
Putnam, F. W., 22, 49, 51, 54, 57

R

Radtke, H. L., 112, 125, 126
Ray, W., 50
Reagor, P. A., 55, 57
Rennick, P. T., 29
Rhue, J. W., 106, 117
Richardson, L. F., 53–57
Roche, S., 20, 21
Ross, C. A., 49
Rossi, E., 26, 27, 29

S

Sanders, B., 55
Sanders, S., 57
Sapp, M., 3, 14, 15, 17, 19, 21, 22, 24, 27, 33, 34, 45, 50, 51, 96, 107, 109, 117, 135
Sarbin, T. R., 10, 33, 101, 106, 118
Sartin-Kirby, R. S., 17, 33, 96
Scharcoff, J., 29
Schilder, P. F., 35
Sexton, M. C., 51
Shallice, T., 117, 120
Sheehan, P. W., 106, 111
Shor, R. E., 34

Silberman, E. K., , 49
Singer, J. L., 16
Sirkin, M. I., 33
Slagle, R. W., 33
Sletten, I., 4
Spanos, N. P., 33, 103, 106, 112, 114, 116, 121, 125, 126
Spiegel, D., 111, 115
Spiegel, H., 106, 111
Stam, H. J., 112
Steinberg, M., 51
Stern, J. A., 4
Straus, H., 42

T

Tan, S., 4
Tellegen, A., 34
Treyens, J. C., 114
Tulis, E., 42
Tyson, G. M., 54

U

Ulett, G. A., 4

V

Vande Creek, L., 56
Van Den Hout, M., 117
Van Gorp. W. G., 29

Venturino, M., 4
Vickery, A. R., 33

W

Wagstaff, G. F., 106
Walker, M. K., 29
Waller, N. G., 22
Watson, R. J., 9
Wegner, D. M., 118, 119
Weishaar, M., 92
Weitzenhoffer, A. M., 10, 111
Wells, G. L., 114
Whalen, J. E., 50
Whalley, L. J., 92
Wheatley, T., 118, 119
Wickless, C., 121
Wilber, C. B., 49
Wilson, S. C., 103, 112
Woody, E. Z., 26, 31, 103, 115, 116, 120, 121

Y

Yant, M., 114
Yapko, M. D., 92

Z

Zamansky, H. S., 120
Zeig, J. K., 29
Zimbardo, P. G., 102, 109, 121

SUBJECT INDEX

A

Abandonment issues, 39
Absorption, 20–21, 60, 79, 102 (see also Imaginative involvement)
Acute stress disorder, 39–40, 54 (see also Dissociative disorders)
   anxiety, 39
   depression, 40
   depersonalization, 39–40
   derealization, 39
   despair, 40
   detachment, 39
   diagnosis criteria, 39–40
   dissociative amnesia, 39–40
   exaggerated startle response, 39
   flashbacks, 39
   hopelessness, 40
   nightmares, 39
   numbing, 39
   symptomology, 39–40
Adaptive regression, 34–35
Adler, A., 14
Age progression, 25, 84–86
Age progression transcript, 84–85
   debriefing, 86
Age regression, 20, 25, 86–87
Age regression transcript, 86–87
   debriefing, 87
Altered state of consciousness, 26–29, 34, 35, 103, 116 (see also Special process theories)
American Society of Clinical Hypnosis (ASCH), 27, 100
Amnesia, 20, 23, 104–5
Amnesic barrier, 31, 116
Amnesic-prone, 104–5, 107, 134–36
   dissociators, 105, 134
Analgesia, 4, 20, 23, 29, 87–89, 121 (see also Pain control)
Anchoring, 29
Anesis, 36–37
Anesthesia, 20, 23
Animal magnetism
   and artificial somnambulism, 11
   –Faria, 10–11
   –Mesmer, 6–7
Anorexia nervosa, 42 (see also Borderline personality disorder)
Anxiety and stress transcript, 90
Anxiety disorders, 39, 89–91
APA's Division 30 definition of hypnosis, 17, 19
Assessment of dissociative disorders in children, 57
Asthma, 4
Attentional resources, 32
Automatic handwriting, 21
Automatic hypnotic responding, 24, 102
Automatic sensory experiences, 24
Automaticity, 13, 15, 102, 115–21
Auto-suggestion, 11–12
Awareness, altered state of, 10, 26–29, 34, 35, 103, 116

B

Barber, Theodore X., 102–6, 134–36
  inductive approach, 102
  motivation and expectancy, 102
  trance and nonstate, 106
Barber's 3-Dimensional Paradigm, 103–6, 134–36
  amnesic-prone, 103, 104–5, 107, 120, 134–36
  fantasy-prone, 103–4, 107, 120, 134–36
  positively-set, 103, 105–7, 120, 134–36
Barber Suggestibility Scale (BSS), 112–13
Baudouin, Charles, 12
Behavior hierarchy arrangements, 30
Behavior initiation theory, 120
Bernheim, Hippolyte, 9–10
Body dysmorphic disorder or dysmorphobia, 41
Borderline personality disorder (BPD), 3, 17, 37–38, 42–45
  abandonment issues, 43
  childlike thinking, 42
  diagnosis criteria, 42–43
  dissociative identity disorders, 42 (see also Dissociative disorders)
  hypnosis applications, 45
  impulsivity, 44
  self-image based on fusing with others, 43–44
  self-mutilation, 44
  suicidal ideation, 44
  symptomology, 43–44
Boundaries
BPD clients, 45
DID clients, 52
  negative sequelae of hypnosis, 98–99
Braid, James, 11, 12, 24

Brain, physiological implications for hypnosis, 31, 108, 116, 135–36
Braun's BASK model, 53
Breuer, Josef, 16
Bulimia, 42 (*see also* Borderline personality disorder)

C

Carleton University Responsiveness to Suggestion Scale (CURSS), 112
Case presentations, 64–66
Case study methodology, 15
Catalepsy, 20, 23
CBH transcript, 76–78, 92
Charcot, Martin Jean, 8, 16, 17, 116
Child abuse and DID, 46, 49–51, 56–57
Child/Adolescent Dissociative Checklist (CADC), 57
Child Dissociative Checklist (CDC), 57
Children's Hypnotic Susceptibility Scale (CHSS), 111
Children's Perceptual Alterations Scale (CPAS), 57
Clairvoyance and hypnosis, 11
Clinical applications
  borderline personality disorder, 45
  phenomena of hypnosis, 37–38
  theories of hypnosis, 18
Clinical interviews with children and liability, 56–57
Cognitive-behavioral hypnosis (CBH), 3, 26–27, 76–78, 92, 112–13
  hypnotizability scales, 112–13
  transcript, 76–78, 92
Cognitive-behavioral theories, 26–27, 32–34, 115
  goal-directed behavior, 33, 34
  role enactment theory, 33
  social psychological, 32–34

sociocognitive, 32–34, 115–7
substantive perspectives of hypnosis, 33–34, 115
Cognitive-behavioral treatments, 19–20, 67, 92
Cognitive relaxation, 37
Combat soldiers and hypnoanalysis, 16, 38 (*see also* PTSD)
   anxiety disorders, 39
   borderline personality disorder, 42
   posttraumatic stress disorder, 3, 16–17, 38, 39
Complexes and dissociated ideations, 16
Consciousness, retraction, 9
Contemporary hypnosis theories and research, 101–33 (*see also* Individuals)
   Barber, Theodore X., 102–6
   Hilgard, E. R., 103
   Sarbin, Theodore, 101–2
   Spanos, N. P., 103
Countertransference, 46, 98
Counting procedures, 67
Conversion disorder, 21, 40–41
Coué, Emile, 11–12
Creative Imagination Scale (CIS), 112
Creativity, 78
   illumination, 78
   incubation, 78
   preparation, 78
   regression in service of ego, 78
   verification/evaluation, 78
Current theories of hypnosis, 26–37, 101–33
   amnesic-prone, 103, 104–5, 107, 120, 134–36
   fantasy-prone, 103–4, 107, 120, 134–36
   nonstate theories, 26, 32–34, 106, 134–36
   positively-set, 103, 105–6, 107, 120, 134–36
   special process theories, 26–29, 34, 106, 134–36
   trance, 106

D

Defense mechanisms and repression, 16, 22
   displacement, 16
   introjection, 16
   overcompensation, 16
   projection, 16
   rationalization, 16
   regression, 16, 34–36, 80
Derealization, 20, 21, 26, 39
Depersonalization, 20, 21, 22, 26, 39–40
Detachment/estrangement, 26, 39–40 (*see also* Acute stress disorder; Depersonalization)
Differential diagnosis and DID, 48
Direct hypnosis, 27–29, 67–69
Direct hypnosis transcript, 67–69
Direct suggestions, 27
Disability, hypnosis and rehabilitation, 96–98
Dissociated control, 31–32
Dissociation, 3, 8, 9, 13, 15, 16–17, 20–22, 102
   and pain relief, 21, 37
   pathology, 9–10, 21–22
   psychoanalysis, 13, 15, 20
   repression, 16–17, 20, 22
   splitting off, 9, 14
Dissociative amnesia, 21, 22, 39–40
Dissociative disorders, 3, 17, 21–22, 39–58
   definition, 39
   diagnostic criteria, 39
   symptomology, 39–40
Dissociative disorders in children, 54–57

amnesic episodes and time loss, 56
assessment, 55–57
screening instruments, 57
symptomology, 54–57
Dissociative Experiences Scale (DES), 21–22, 51
Dissociative fugues, 21, 22
Dissociative hypnosis, 67
Dissociative identity disorder (DID), 3, 17, 21, 22, 37, 45–54
amnesia patterns, 46
child abuse, 46
description, 46–48
diagnostic criteria, 47, 49–50
differential diagnosis, 48
dissociation hypnosis transcript, 83–84
gender differences, 47–48
hypnotic fusion technique transcript, 82–83
memory and identity disturbances, 46–48
personalities existence, 46–48 (see also Integration of personalities)
treatment, 49–54
Dissociation theories, 14, 29–32
dissociated control theory, 31–32, 116, 120
neodissociation, 30–31, 116, 120
Dissociation transcript, 83–84
Dream analysis, 14

E

Effect size measures, 19–20
Ego, 14, 30, 31, 35, 78–79, 116
attention and absorption, 79, 102
ego activity and free will, 78
ego passivity and coping inability, 78
ego receptivity and reality orientation, 79
ego-strengthening induction, 91
general reality orientation, 79
self-hypnosis and concentrated attention, 79
Ego-strengthening induction transcript, 91
Emotionality, 89
Erickson, M. H., 14, 27
Ericksonian hypnosis, 12, 27–29, 69
Executive ego, 30, 31, 103, 116 (see also Neodissociation)
Expectancy theory, 20, 102
Expectations, 19, 20, 35, 102

F

Fantasy-prone, 3, 21, 102, 103–4, 107, 134–46
Faria, Abbé, 10–11
Franklin, Benjamin, 7
Free association, 14, 17
Freud, Sigmund, 8, 13–18
overview of integration of theories, 15
phases of psychoanalysis, 13–15
repression, 16–17
Fromm, Erika, 35, 45, 78–79
attention and absorption, 79, 102
structure and content, 79
ego activity and free will, 78
ego passivity and coping inability, 78
ego receptivity and reality orientation, 79
general reality orientation, 79
hypnotic relaxation, 78
psychoanalysis and hypnosis, 78–79
regression in service of the ego, 78
self-hypnosis and concentrated

attention, 79
Frontal lobe dysfunction, 31, 108, 116, 135–36
Fugues, 21

G

General Dissociation Scale (GDS), 22, 51
General Reality Orientation (GRO), 79
Goal-directed behavior, 33, 34 (*see also* Cognitive-behavioral theories)
Guillotin, Joseph, 7

H

Hadfield, J. A., 16, 17
Hallucinations, 20, 25, 42, 44, 48, 54–55, 105
Hand levitation hypnotic screening test, 61, 63
    debriefing, 64
    induction script, 62
Handclasp hypnotic screening test, 61
    debriefing, 62
    induction script, 62
Harvard Group Scale of Hypnotic Susceptibility Form A (HGSHS:A), 110
Hell, Father Maximillian, 6
Hilgard, E. R., 103
    altered-state theory, 103
    dissociated control theory, 103
Hyperamnesia, 20, 23, 79
Hyperesthesia, 20, 23
Hypersuggestibility, 10
Hypnoanalysis, 17 (*see also* Hadfield)
Hypnosis
    and anxiety/stress, 89–91
    –BPD, 45
    –DID, 53
    –ego strengthening, 91–92
    –memory, 10, 114–15
    –pain control, 4, 37, 67, 87–89
    –rehabilitation, 96–98
    –trait/skill models, 10–11, 121
    –weight loss, 95–96
    clinical applications, 18, 37–38
    cognitive-behavioral approaches, 32–34
    direct v. indirect, 27, 67, 69
    negative sequelae, 98–99
    overview of process, 4–5, 19–38
    relaxation inductions, 36–37, 96–98
    response expectations, 20, 102, 117
    screening tests, 61–64
    tailoring to client, 28 (*see also* Erickson)
Hypnosis, automaticity, involuntariness, and nonvolitional responding, 13, 15, 30–31, 102, 115–21
    conditions for behavioral action, 115
Hypnosis, transcripts
    age regression, 84–85
    debriefing, 86
    anxiety/stress, 90
    cognitive-behavioral (CBH), 76–78
    dissociation, 83–84
    debriefing, 84
    ego-strengthening induction, 91
    debriefing, 92
    fusion technique for DID, 82–83
    debriefing, 83
    hand levitation hypnotic screening test, 63
    debriefing, 64
    handclasp hypnotic screening test, 62
    debriefing, 63
    ingredients, 66–67
    pain control, 88–89

debriefing, 89
psychodynamic hypnosis, 80–81
  debriefing, 81
smoking, 94–95
  debriefing, 95
unipolar depression, 92–93
  debriefing, 93
weight loss, 95–96
  debriefing, 96
Hypnotic
depth, 109–11
handclasp hypnotic screening test, 62
regression and intellectual functioning, 36
relaxation, 36–37, 78–79, 96–98 (*see also* Relaxation theory)
response expectations, 20, 102, 117
responsiveness, 10–11, 108–9
suggestion, 10, 11, 106–8
susceptibility, 24, 61
Hypnotic experience, description (DHE), 126
Hypnotic Induction Profile (HIP), 111
Hypnotic involuntariness theory, 117
Hypnotic screening tests, 61–64
  hand levitation test, 61
  handclasp test, 61
Hypnotic survey (HS), 123–26
Hypnotic treatment, 59–100
  client preparation, 59–61
Hypnotizability
  correlates, 61
  factorial design, 106–7
  phenomena, 20, 108–11, 134–36
Hypnotizability measures and theoretical perspectives, 4, 113
Hypnotizability scales, 4, 47, 108–11
Hypnotizability scales reflecting cognitive-behavioral orientation, 4
Hypochondriasis, 41
Hysteria, 6–8, 17, 40
  Briquets Syndrome, 40
Charcot, 8, 17, 116
Freud, 13–17
Janet, 9, 17, 116
Mesmer, 6–7, 17
somatoform disorders, 3, 17, 38, 40
  diagnosis criteria, 40
  trauma association, 8, 16, 116

I

Ideomotor and ideosensory exploration, 20, 24, 61, 79, 115, 135
Imaginative involvement, 3, 12, 20, 61, 103 (*see also* Absorption)
Implications for pain control, 4, 37, 67, 87–89
Indirect hypnosis, 27–29, 67, 69–76
Indirect hypnosis transcript, 69–76
  debriefing, 76
Indirect Hypnotic Susceptibility Scale Wexler-Alman, 113, 114
Indirect Hypnotic Susceptibility Scale (WAIHSS), 113
Indirect suggestions, 10, 11, 27, 28
Induction scripts (*see also* Hypnosis, transcripts)
Ingredients of hypnosis transcripts, 62, 66–67
  counting procedures, 67
  preinduction talk, 66
  progressive relaxation, 66–67
  termination suggestions, 67
Inhibition, 31
Integration of DID personalities, 49–54
Interactive-phenomenological theories, 34
International Society for the Study of Dissociation (ISSD), 49, 51, 100
  treatment guidelines, 49–53
Intrapsychic nature of psychic energy, 15
Involuntariness, 103

Subject Index

Ironic process theory, 118–19

J

Janet, Pierre, 9, 16, 17, 116
Jung, Carl, 14

L

Lavoisier, Antoine, 7
Liébault, 9–10
Lucid sleep, 11 (*see also* Faria)

M

Magnetic forces and psychological disorders, 6–7
Marquis de Puységur, 11
Measures of hypnotic responding, 10–11, 108–9
Memory and hypnosis, 10, 114–15
Memory reconstruction, 56, 114–15
Mentation, 14
Mesmer and animal magnetism, 6–7
Mesmerism
    Braid and nervous sleep, 12
    Charcot, 8
    Janet, 9
Mesmer, 6–7
Mesmer, Anton Franz, 6–7, 17
Meta-analyses, 19–20
Migraine headaches, 4
Motoric relaxation, 37
Multiple personality disorder (see Dissociative identity disorder)
Multiple sclerosis, 8
Multilevel communication, 28

N

Nancy School, 9–10, 11–12
Nash, Michael, 80–82
Naturalistic hypnosis, 27, 69
Neoclassical conditioning theory, 117
Neodissociation, 30–31
Neurolinguistic programming (NLP), 29–30
    anchoring, 29
    reframing, 29
Neuropsychological dissociative phenomena, 21
Nonhypnotic relaxation, 36–37
Nonstate theorists, 26–27, 32–34, 106
Nonvolitional, 13, 15, 30–31, 102, 115–21
Numbing, 39

O

Overview of dissociative identity disorder (DID), 45–54

P

Pain control, 4, 37, 67
    direct hypnosis, 67
    implication of hypnois, 87–89
Pain control transcript, 88–89
Pain disorder, 41
Paralelsus, Philippus, 6
Permissive hypnosis, 27
Phenomena of hypnosis (see Barber's 3-dimensional paradigm)
    amnesic-prone, 104–5, 107, 134–36
    fantasy-prone, 103–4, 107, 134–36
    positively-set clients, 19–38, 105–7, 134–36
Possible negative sequelae of hypnosis, 98–99
Postfusion treatment, 53
    Braun's BASK model, 53
Posttraumatic stress disorder (PTSD), 3, 16–17, 38, 39, 54
    anxiety disorders, 39

borderline personality disorder, 42
diagnosis criteria, 39–40
dissociative identity disorder, 46
symptomology, 39–40 (see also Acute stress disorder)
Preparation of client for hypnosis, 59–61
education re modality, 60
absorption, 60, 102
adjunctive procedure, 60, 115
client's misconceptions, 60
imagery and relaxation, 60
self-hypnosis, 60, 116
types of hypnosis, 60
uses of hypnosis, 60
psychotherapy skills, 60–61
Preinduction talk, 66
Primary process thinking, 14
dreams, 14
nonlogic and id principle, 14
poetry, 14
psychosis, 14
Progressive relaxation, 67
Pseudocyesis, 41
Psychic energy, 15
Psychoanalysis and hypnosis, 13–15, 16–17, 45
BPD and boundaries, 45
separation-individuation process, 45
Psychoanalysis and repression, 16–17, 20
Psychoanalysis, Freud's phases, 13–15
definitions of terminology, 13
Psychodynamic hypnosis transcript, 80–81
debriefing, 81
Psychodynamic orientation to hypnosis, 36, 67
Psychological disorders and uses of hypnosis, 3
Psychological dissociative phenomena, 21
Psychological regression, 13, 15, 34–36
Psychotherapy goals and hypnosis, 3, 19–38, 45
Psychotherapy skills, 60–61
Level I, 60
Level II, 61

R

Reframing, 29
Regression, 13, 15, 34–36, 80 (see also Psychological regression)
adaptive, 34–35
revivification, 35
temporal, 35, 80
topographic, 35, 80
Regressive hypnosis, 67
Rehabilitation hypnosis, 96–98
Relaxation theory of hypnosis, 34, 36–37, 78–79, 96–96
anesis, 36–37
cognitive, 37, 78
disability and rehabilitation, 96–98
ego-modulated relaxation of defensive barriers, 78
impact of mechanism, 37
motoric, 37
Repression, 15, 16–17, 20, 22
dissociation, 16, 20, 22
Freudian theory, 16–17
Research instruments, 121–32
Description of Hypnotic Experience (DHE), 126
General Dissociation Scale (GDS), 127–32
Hypnotic Survey (HS), 123–26
Vividness of Imagination Scale (VIS), 121–23
Research, summaries and findings of contemporary theories, 106–33
Response expectancy theory, 117

Subject Index

Role enactment theory, 33

S

Sarbin, Theodore, 101–2
   role taking theory, 102
   social psychological behavior, 101
Schemata theory, 117–18
Schizophrenia, affective disorders, BPD, 42–45
Schizophrenia and DID, 48
Screening instruments for dissociative disorders with children, 57
Secondary process thinking, 14
   ego and reality principle, 14, 34–36
Self-hypnosis, 21, 103, 116
Self-image based on fusing with others, 43–44
Self-mutilation, 44
Separation-individuation process for BPD, 45
Sexual relations, 98–99
   transference/countertransference, 98–99
Sleep, lucid, 11 (see also Faria)
Sleep, nervous, 12 (see also Braid)
Smoking, 93–95
Smoking cessation transcript, 94–95
   debriefing, 95
Social-cognition theories, 26–27, 31–32
   sociocognitive, 32–34, 115–7
Social psychological, 26–27
Society for Clinical and Experimental Hypnosis (SCEH), 100
Sociophenomenological theories, 26–27, 32–38
Somatoform disorders, 3, 17, 38, 40, 54 (see also Hysteria)
   diagnosis criteria, 40
Somnambulism, 24

Spanos, N. P., 103
   goal-directed fantasies, 103
   strategic role enactment, 103
Special process theories of hypnosis, 26–29, 34
Splitting off, 9, 14
Stanford Hypnotic Clinical Scale (SHCS), 111
Stanford Hypnotic Clinical Scale for Children (SHCSC), 111
Stanford Profile Scale of Hypnotic Ability (SPS:I&II), 111
Stanford Scale of Hypnotic Susceptibility (SHSS), 110
Startle response, exaggerated, 39–40
Stern, Adolph, 42
Structured Clinical Interview for DSM–IV–R, 51
Suggestibility, 10, 11, 12, 102 (see also Auto-suggestion)
   difference between suggesstions, suggestibility, 12
Suicidal ideation, 44
Sullivan, H. S., 14
Suppression, 22–23
Surgeries and hypnosis, 4

T

Tellegen Absorption Scale (TAS), 21
Temporal regression, 35 (see also Regression)
Termination suggestions, 67
Therapeutic suggestion, 9–10 (see also Liébault)
Time distortion, 20, 25
Topographic regression, 35 (see also Regression)
Traditional hypnosis, 4
Trance, 26–29, 34, 35, 79, 102, 103, 106
Transference relationship, 35–36, 98
Trauma, 3, 16–17, 116

anxiety disorders, 39
borderline personality disorder, 42
child abuse and DID, 49–51
diagnosis criteria, 39–40
posttraumatic stress disorder (PTSD), 3, 16–17, 38, 39
Treatment of DID, 49–54

U

Unconscious information, reaching via hypnosis, 4, 12, 13
Unipolar depression, 92,
hypnosis transcript, 92–93
Universal spirit, 6–7
Uses of hypnosis, 3–5

V

Vividness of Imagination Scale (VIS), 121–23
Volitional activity, 78

W

Warts, 4
Waterloo-Standard Group Scale of Hypnotic Susceptibility (WSGS), 110
Weight loss transcript, 95–96
Worry, 89

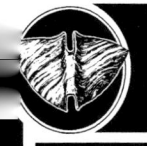

Charles C Thomas
PUBLISHER • LTD.

2600 South First Street
Springfield, IL 62704

NEW *from Charles C Thomas, Publisher!*

- Feldman, Saul—**MANAGED BEHAVIORAL HEALTH SERVICES: Perspectives and Practice.** '02, 458 pp. (7 x 10), 6 il., 10 tables.

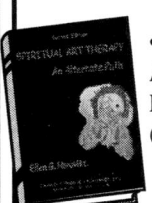

- Horovitz, Ellen G.—**SPIRITUAL ART THERAPY: An Alternate Path. (2nd Ed.)** '02, 246 pp. (7 x 10), 47 il., 2 tables.

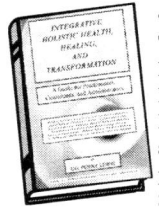

- Lewis, Penny—**INTEGRATIVE HOLISTIC HEALTH, HEALING, AND TRANSFORMATION: A Guide for Practitioners, Consultants, and Administrators.** '02, 366 pp. (7 x 10), 31 il., $69.95, hard, $49.95, paper.

- Lathom-Radocy, Wanda B.—**PEDIATRIC MUSIC THERAPY.** '02, 360 pp. (7 x 10), $76.95, hard, $52.95, paper.

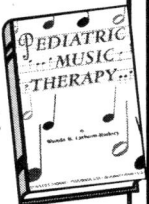

- Arrington, Doris Banowsky—**HOME IS WHERE THE ART IS: An Art Therapy Approach to Family Therapy.** '01, 294 pp. (7 x 10), 109 il. (1 in color), 18 tables, $61.95, hard, $42.95, paper.

- Landy, Robert J.—**HOW WE SEE GOD AND WHY IT MATTERS: A Multicultural View Through Children's Drawings and Stories.** '01, 234 pp. (8 1/2 x 11), 55 il. (40 in color), $58.95, hard, $41.95, paper.

- Landy, Robert J.—**NEW ESSAYS IN DRAMA THERAPY: Unfinished Business.** '01, 250 pp. (8 1/2 x 11), 15 il. (14 in color), 4 tables, $57.95, hard, $36.95, paper.

- Spring, Dee—**IMAGE AND MIRAGE: Art Therapy with Dissociative Clients.** '01, 288 pp. (7 x 10), 49 il., $55.95, hard, $38.95, paper.

- Stepney, Stella A.—**ART THERAPY WITH STUDENTS AT RISK: Introducing Art Therapy into an Alternative Learning Environment for Adolescents.** '01, 140 pp. (8 1/2 x 11), 14 il. (14 in color), 5 tables, $42.95, hard, $25.95, paper.

- Lewis, Penny & David Read Johnson—**CURRENT APPROACHES IN DRAMA THERAPY.** '00, 502 pp. (7 x 10), 23 il., 1 table, $89.95, hard, $59.95, paper.

Contact us to order books or a free catalog with over 811 titles

Call 1-800-258-8980 or 1-217-789-8980 or Fax 1-217-789-9130
Complete catalog available at www.ccthomas.com • books@ccthomas.com

Books sent on approval • Shipping charges: $6.95 U.S. / Outside U.S., actual shipping fees will be charged
Prices subject to change without notice